Diversity, Gender Equity and Inclusion in Critical Care and Perioperative Medicine

Vojislava Neskovic • Francesca Rubulotta
Editors

Diversity, Gender Equity and Inclusion in Critical Care and Perioperative Medicine

A New Guidance for Team Excellence

Springer

Editors
Vojislava Neskovic
Clinic for Anesthesia and Critical Care,
Faculty of Medicine MMA
Military Medical Academy
Belgrade, Serbia

Francesca Rubulotta
Department of Critical Care Medicine
McGill University Health Centre
Montreal, QC, Canada

ISBN 978-3-031-86285-4 ISBN 978-3-031-86286-1 (eBook)
https://doi.org/10.1007/978-3-031-86286-1

This Springer imprint is published by the registered company Springer Nature Switzerland AG
The registered company address is: Gewerbestrasse 11, 6330 Cham, Switzerland

This book is dedicated to Jannicke Melin-Olsen.

Foreword

Why should anyone bother to read a book on gender equity and diversity in the 2020s? Two hundred and forty years since the first known scientific society for women was founded, are we not done with the Redstockings movement of the 1970s? Is it not time to concentrate on "real" problems in medicine and the society as whole?

Complacency is a dangerous state, as it leaves us ignorant of our blind spots and prevents us from development. This book shows us that many of those blind spots still are present.

Superiors may have a seemingly good reason when they hire a male and not a female and why men get higher salaries than women doing similar jobs. Researchers and congress organisers who end up with all-men groups are "not looking for sexes, but only for the best research partners and speakers at conferences". When parents decide who will be more home with the children, they give perfectly sound arguments that "just in our case, it is better for the mother", but fail to acknowledge that the pattern of most parents thinking the same illustrate that this is a structural issue.

It is easy to understand why clinical trials including volunteers would have proportionally higher representation of young men at a time that most medical students were men. It is understandable that in societies that were white male dominated, one had to go outside the box to grasp the idea that "the norm" does not give the full picture.

This book helps us see more of that picture and beyond. The authors provide both theoretical background, create awareness and give us practical advice on how to improve. The authors illustrate that although we are equally valuable, all humans are not created the same. We must be aware of in all walks of life, including professional, academic and personal life. This goes for age, sex and gender, ethnical and cultural background, life conditions and prosperity, and other factors.

"Bias" and "preconception" are normal psychological properties. They serve us well, as we need them to create some order of all the impressions that we receive every second. But if we are unaware of the mechanisms and side effects they possess, then we risk making the wrong judgement and take the wrong decisions.

Equity and diversity in intensive care and perioperative medicine is the focus of the book, but the mechanisms and factors that are described are valid in other fields of medicine and society, as well.

A valuable aspect of this book is that although the main spotlight is on sex and gender, it includes a wide range of diversity topics, be it in science, education, research, personal and global factors. Sex and gender balance serves as example of several other types of inequities in life and medicine. An important message is that we should consider diversity, not only to be nice to others but also to ensure better treatment for our patients and to create better private and professional lives in a balanced society.

Only when each of us and the society are aware of these blind spots can we learn and improve. The authors of this book help us in the right direction.

Past President World Federation of Societies of Anaesthesiologists
London, UK
jannicke@mellin.no

Jannicke Melin-Olsen

Foreword

I am thrilled to introduce a preface for a forthcoming book that delves into the crucial topic of gender equity in the field of medicine, particularly focusing on training, role models, and the definition of gender equity and diversity in critical care and perioperative settings. This book aims to shed light on the various aspects of gender disparities within the medical realm and propose solutions to bridge these gaps.

Different aspects will be discussed: the book will explore the implications of gender equity and diversity in clinical trials and how new funding policies can influence healthcare outcomes. It will delve into the realm of women's health beyond maternal care, uncovering the gender inequalities that persist in health care and their impact on patient outcomes, and will provide insights into the perioperative management and care of critically ill pregnant patients, highlighting the importance of gender-sensitive healthcare practices.

The book will also discuss non-pregnancy-related emergencies in critically ill and surgical female patients, shedding light on the unique challenges they face in healthcare settings, and will explore the role of patient satisfaction as an outcome in patient-centered care and the importance of diversity in enhancing healthcare experiences. Finally, the book will address the underrepresentation of gender and minorities in critical care and perioperative medicine, calling for greater inclusivity in the healthcare workforce, providing a cross-section of the current scenarios and international actions being taken to promote gender equity and diversity in healthcare.

This work delves into the implementation of gender equity and diversity in curricula related to critical care and perioperative medicine, emphasizing the importance of inclusive educational practices with the aim to improve well-being and achieving success in critical care, anesthesia, and critical care settings through gender-sensitive approaches. The book wraps up with a discussion on preventing harassment to enhance team well-being and patient safety in healthcare environments, underscoring the need for a supportive and inclusive workplace culture. This book serves as a comprehensive guide for healthcare professionals, educators, and policymakers to foster gender equity and diversity in medicine, ultimately striving toward a more inclusive and equitable healthcare system.

I strongly believe this was really needed in the current medical community and will lead to improvement of current reality and gender balance.

Anaesthesia and Intensive Care, IRCCS Policlinico San Martino, Genova, Italy Chiara Robba

Chair of the Neurointensive Care Section of European Society of Intensive Care Medicine, Genova, Italy

Direttore Sds Medicina del dolore e Cure Palliative, Genova, Italy

Preface

"Each one of us has a different idea of who we are."
Luigi Pirandello

The editors are proud to present the first edition of this book on diversity, equity, and inclusion (DEI) in perioperative and critical care medicine. Recent years have highlighted specific interests within this field, illustrating both its relevance and urgency. Perioperative and critical care medicine face unique challenges, not only due to a lack of diversity but also concerning the well-being and professional growth of medical professionals from varied backgrounds. Patients also experience significant challenges in these areas. Sex- and gender-informed medicine is an emerging paradigm in clinical practice and research, examining how sex and gender influence all aspects of the disease process, from risk assessment to symptom presentation and treatment response. Despite advancements, many knowledge gaps persist, underscoring the need for ongoing research and dialogue.

Our journey to writing this book began at the Euroanesthesia 2022 Congress in Milan, where the Gender Equity Committee of the European Society of Anaesthesiology and Intensive Care hosted sessions dedicated to equity and women's health. This event served as a catalyst for our collaboration, which has focused on empowering women through initiatives such as the International Women in Intensive and Critical Care Medicine Network (iWIN). Together, we have worked to strengthen the platform for women in the field, fostering networking, sponsorship, mentorship, and advocacy to address the challenges women face and improve opportunities in anesthesiology and critical care medicine.

By leveraging our global network, we were able to engage contributors from across the world, culminating in the assembly of all chapters in Catania, Sicily. What began in Milan has now become a project enriched by diverse global perspectives, reflecting the experiences and origins of the editors. This journey has come full circle, with both its beginning and completion in Italy, a testament to the power of collaboration and shared vision.

We believe that this is the call for interaction and action in building improved working environment and well-being for professionals, and human rights and justice for all patients regardless to their differences. The book's structure encourages readers to rethink various topics, with chapters addressing crucial questions faced by both professionals and patients in today's world.

The contributions come from a distinguished group of experts and advocates in DEI, representing a wide range of professional interests and cultural backgrounds, as well as diverse races, religions, and a balanced mix of men and women from all continents. The aim was to minimize bias and reflect a wide range of viewpoints, enriching the discussion with a global perspective on critical issues. We are grateful for the enthusiasm and dedication of our contributors. Our hope is that this book will inspire a cultural shift toward fairness, justice, and improved standards of care in perioperative, critical care medicine, and beyond.

Belgrade, Serbia — Vojislava Neskovic
Montreal, QC, Canada — Francesca Rubulotta

The original version of this book has been revised. A foreword by Dr. Jannicke Mellin-Olsen and a Dedication from Editors has been included in the book. An error in the last sentence on page xv and contributors' list on the pages xvi-xix have been updated in 'About the Editors and Contributors' section.

Contents

About the Editors and Contributors

Editors

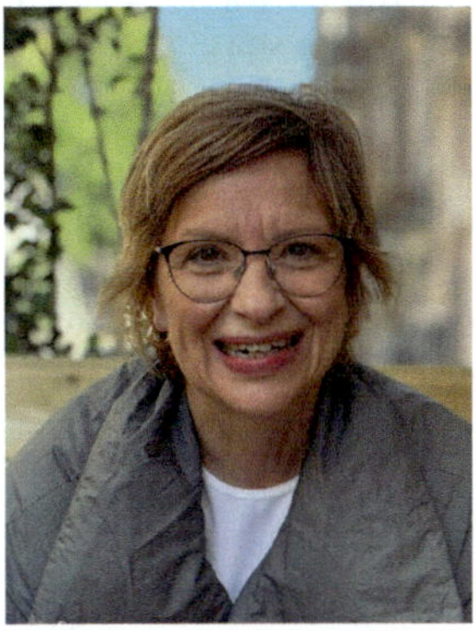

Vojislava Neskovic is an Associate Professor in Anaesthesia and Intensive Care at the Military Medical Academy in Belgrade, Serbia, where she also teaches at the Medical Faculty. She is an active member of the European Association of Cardiothoracic Anaesthesiology and Intensive Care (EACTAIC) Thoracic Subcommittee, the European Society of Anaesthesiology and Intensive Care (ESAIC) Teach the Teachers Masterclass Faculty and Committee, and serves as an examiner for the European Diploma of Anaesthesia and Intensive Care (EDAIC). Previously, she served as Chair of Department of Anaesthesia and Intensive Care at the Institute of Cardiovascular Diseases in Sremska Kamenica. Dr. Neskovic was the inaugural Chair of the European Society of Anaesthesiology and Intensive Care (ESAIC) Gender Equity Committee and has also held the position of President of the Serbian Association of Anaesthesiologists and Intensivists. Outside her professional life, she is married, has two adult daughters, a film director and a physician, and a dog named Badi.

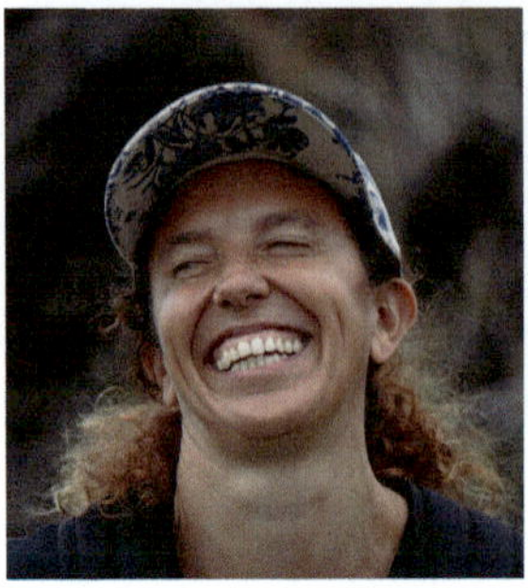

Francesca Rubulotta has a PhD in medicine and a Master in Business Administration. She has over 30 years of experience in Medicine and innovation. Dr. Rubulotta is an Associate Professor of Anaesthesia, Critical Care Medicine, and pain medicine at the University of Catania, Italy, and is the Director of the residency program. She was an Associate Professor at McGill University and the Chief of the Critical Care Program at the Montreal General Hospital and the Royal Victoria Hospital, McGill University Health Centers, Québec, Canada. She was the inaugural Chair of the Department of Critical Care Medicine at the McGill University Campus in Montreal, Québec, Canada. Dr. Rubulotta was a consultant for 12 years at Charing Cross and St Mary's Hospital, NHS Trust, and Honorary Senior Clinical Lecturer in Anaesthesia and Intensive Care Medicine at Imperial College Medical School in London, UK. Dr. Rubulotta is the chair of the non-profit organization International Women in Intensive and Critical Care Network (iWIN, www.iwin-ideal.com). Dr. Rubulotta is one of the organizers of the World Day of the Critical Lung.

Contributors

Alice Agostinelli Barts and The London School of Medicine and Dentistry, London, UK

Maham Jawaid Ahmad Department of Critical Care Medicine, Ziauddin University, Karachi, Pakistan

Antonio Artigas Intensive Care Department, Corporacion Sanitaria Universitaria Parc Tauli. Institut d'Investigació i Innovació Parc Tauli (I3PT). Autonomous University of Barcelona, Sabadell, Spain

Raffaele Aspide IRCCS Istituto delle Scienze Neurologiche di Bologna – Anesthesia and Intensive Care Unit, Bologna, Italy

Suzana Atanasoski University Medicine Zurich, University of Zurich, Zurich, Switzerland

Denise Battaglini Anesthesia and Intensive Care, IRCCS Ospedale Policlinico San Martino, Genoa, Italy

Beatrice Beck-Schimmer Institute of Anaesthesiology, University Hospital Zurich, University of Zurich, Zurich, Switzerland

Joana Berger-Estilita Chair of the Education and Training Committee, ESAIC, FMH für Anästhesiologie und Intensivmedizin, Consultant in Anaesthesiology and Intensive Care Salemspital, Hirslanden Medical Group, Bern, Switzerland
Scientific Collaborator, Institute for Medical Education, University of Bern, Bern, Switzerland

Federico Bilotta Department of Anesthesiology, Intensive care and pain management, "Sapienza" University of Rome, Rome, Italy

Nicolas Brogly Anesthesia and Reanimation, Hospital Universitario Gregorio Marañón, Madrid, Spain

María Cruz Martín Delgado Intensive Care Unit, Hospital Universitario 12 Octubre, Madrid, Spain

Gauri Raman Gangakhedkar Department of Anesthesiology, Critical Care and Pain, Tata Memorial Hospital, Homi Bhabha National Institute, Mumbai, India

Naeha Geogy University of Washington, Seattle, WA, USA

Fernando Gilsanz Real Academia Nacional de Medicina. Universidad Autónoma de Madrid, Facultad de Medicina UAM, Madrid, Spain

Mia Gisselbaek Division of Anesthesiology, Department of Anesthesiology, Pharmacology, Intensive Care, and Emergency Medicine, Geneva University Hospitals and Faculty of Medicine, University of Geneva, Geneva, Switzerland
Unit of Development and Research in Medical Education (UDREM), Faculty of Medicine, University of Geneva, Geneva, Switzerland

Pascale Gruber The Royal Marsden NHS Foundation Trust, London, UK

Emilia Guasch Anesthesia and Reanimation Department. WFSA obstetric anesthesia subcommittee chair., Hospital Universitario Fundación Jiménez Díaz, Madrid, Spain

Judith Gutiérrez Gutiérrez Intensive Care Unit, Hospital Universitario 12 Octubre, Madrid, Spain

Bethany Gwyther Whittington Health NHS Trust, London, UK

Olfa Hamzaoui Service de Médecine Intensive-Réanimation Polyvalente, Hôpital Robert Debré, Centre hospitalo-universitaire de Reims, Reims, France
Unité HERVI Hémostase et Remodelage Vasculaire Post-Ischémie-EA 3801, Université de Reims, Reims, France

Madiha Hashmi Department of Critical Care Medicine, Ziauddin University, Karachi, Pakistan
CCM Fellowship & MD Programme, Ziauddin Group of Hospitals, Visiting Faculty, Aga Khan University, Karachi, Pakistan
Honorary Physician MORU, Bangkok, Secretary Faculty of CCM, Bangkok, Thailand

Alexandra M. Hogan Salisbury Hospital Foundation Trust, Salisbury, UK
School of Health Sciences, University of Southampton, Salisbury, UK

Cristina Honorato-Cia Department of Anaesthesia and Critical Care, Clínica Universidad de Navarra, Pamplona, Spain

Aasma Khan Department of Critical Care Medicine, Ziauddin University, Karachi, Pakistan

Angelly Martinez Clin Ultrasound Clinical Governance Lead Organ Donation Specialist CICM SOT GCHS Intensive Care Unit, Robina, QLD, Australia

Luciana Mascia Dipartimento di Medicina Sperimentale, University of Salento, Lecce, Italy

Sheila Nainan Myatra Department of Anesthesiology, Critical Care and Pain, Tata Memorial Hospital, Homi Bhabha National Institute, Mumbai, India

Prof Vojislava Neskovic, MD, PhD Clinic for Anesthesia and Critical Care, Faculty of Medicine MMA, Military Medical Academy, Belgrade, Serbia

Ornella Piazza Department of Medicine, University of Salerno, Salerno, Italy

Katarzyna Prus Department of Neurology, University Clinical Hospital No 4 - Medical University of Lublin, Lublin, Poland

Jordi Rello Universitat Internacional de Catalunya, Barcelona, Spain
CRIPS Research Group-Vall d'Hebrón Institute Research Ps Vall d'Hebron 119, AMI– 14a Planta, Barcelona, Spain

Emilio Rodriguez-Ruiz Intensive Care Medicine Department, University Clinic Hospital of Santiago de Compostela (CHUS), Santiago de Compostela, Spain

Simulation, Life Support, and Intensive Care Research Unit (SICRUS), Health Research Institute of Santiago de Compostela (IDIS), Santiago de Compostela, Spain

Silvia De Rosa Centre for Medical Sciences-CISMed, University of Trento, Trento, Italy

Anesthesia and Intensive Care, Santa Chiara Regional Hospital, APSS, Trento, Italy

Prof Francesca Rubulotta Director of the Residency Program in Anesthesia and Critical Care Medicine, MD, PhD, MBA Department of Anaesthesia and Critical Care, Ospedale Gaspare Rodolico, Catania, Italy
International Women in Intensive and Critical Care Medicine, iWIN ETS, Catania, Italy

Charlotte Salmon Gandonnière Médecine Intensive Réanimation, CHRU de Tours, Tours, France
INSERM CIC 1415, CHRU de Tours, Tours, France
FEMMIR group for the SRLF Trial group, Tours, France

Filippo Sanfilippo Department of Anesthesia and Intensive care – Policlinico Rodolico San Marco University hospital Catania, Catania, CT, Italy

Cristina Santonocito Department of Anesthesia and Intensive Care – CAST Rodolico San Marco University Hospital, Catania, Italy

Sukhada Savarkar Department of Anesthesiology, Critical Care and Pain, Tata Memorial Hospital, Homi Bhabha National Institute, Mumbai, India

Sarah Saxena Department of Anesthesiology, Helora, Mons, Belgium
Department of Surgery, UMons, Research Institute for Health Sciences and Technology, University of Mons, Mons, Belgium

Martin Schläpfer Institute of Anaesthesiology, University Hospital Zurich, Institute of Physiology, University of Zurich, Zurich, Switzerland

Deeya Sharma University of Washington, Seattle, WA, USA

Fiona Melanie Uhor, University of Bern, Bern, Switzerland
Faculty of Medicine, University of Ljubljana, Ljubljana, Slovenia

Luigi La Via Department of Anesthesia and Intensive Care, University Hospital Policlinico G. Rodolico-San Marco, Catania, Italy

Marcela Vizcaychipi Imperial College London, London, UK
Chelsea & Westminster NHS Foundation Trust, London, UK

Ulrike Weber-Stadlbauer University Medicine Zurich, University of Zurich, Zurich, Switzerland

Marko Zdravkovic Faculty of Medicine, University of Maribor, Maribor, Slovenia
Department of Anesthesiology, Intensive Care and Pain Management, University Medical Centre Maribor, Maribor, Slovenia

List of Videos

Part I

Introduction

Definition of the Concept of Gender Equity and Diversity in Critical Care and Perioperative Settings

1

Vojislava Neskovic and Francesca Rubulotta

1.1 Introduction

The most relevant questions that the reader asks at the beginning of every book are why this book is written and the reason for reading it.

At the beginning of this book, the question is why we discuss gender equality, equity, diversity, and inclusion in the perioperative and critical care setting. Why are they important? Or are we able to recognize inequality, stereotypes and bias, lack of different opportunities which influence professional development or disparity of medical care and different outcomes in this environment?

Initially, we need to set the common ground and introduce terms and targets that will be discussed in this book.

The basic definition of gender equality is that all individuals (patients, families, professionals, and healthcare workers) are free to develop their abilities and make choices without limitations imposed by gender rules. Equity goes further: all individuals do not have the same starting point and adjustments to the imbalances should be made to fulfil personal abilities and choices. Equality and equity guarantee fairness, justice, and basic human rights [1]. The final goal is not to become the same; the rights and opportunities of everyone should not depend on gender [1]. The concept of intersectionality explains how gender, age, race, ethnicity, class, sexuality, religion, disability, weight, and physical appearance, migration not only between

V. Neskovic (✉)
Clinic for Anesthesia and Critical Care, Faculty of Medicine MMA, Military Medical Academy, Belgrade, Serbia

F. Rubulotta
Department of Anaesthesia and Critical Care, Ospedale Gaspare Rodolico, Catania, Italy

International Women in Intensive and Critical Care Medicine, iWIN ETS, Catania, Italy
e-mail: francesca.rubulotta@unict.it

V. Neskovic, F. Rubulotta (eds.), *Diversity, Gender Equity and Inclusion in Critical Care and Perioperative Medicine*,
https://doi.org/10.1007/978-3-031-86286-1_1

different countries but within one, may overlap and create different modes of discrimination or privilege. Usually, it is not only gender that creates unfairness and inequity [2].

Gender bias and stereotypes have negative effects on all people and communities. They are not a 'women's thing' but relate to a culture that does not tolerate diversity. Nonetheless, inequalities appear to have a greater impact on women, and it is easier to recognize them by looking at gender compared to other variables. Gender equality and equity are not just "technical things" either. They will not be solved by simply counting gender at different positions and ticking the boxes. It is a highly political issue that requires a substantial level of social consensus to move forward [1].

Diversity is more complex to define, and, in this book, it refers to a variety of identities of every party within the perioperative and critical care environment. Diversity determines the need for inclusion and equal access to opportunities and resources for all: both patients and healthcare professionals.

In 2015, all United Nations Member States adopted the 17 Sustainable Development Goals (SDGs) to achieve a better future for all people [3]. This was an urgent call to action to address the global challenges we face to bring peace and justice. Ideally, goals have been projected to be accomplished by 2030. Achieving gender equality and empowering all women and girls is placed fifth between ending poverty, and hunger, ensuring good education, and clean water, addressing climate change, and protecting life on earth [4]. Unfortunately, according to the available indicators, the world is not on track to achieve gender equality by the predicted deadline. At the current rate of improvement, it will take 285 years to close gaps in legal protection and remove discriminatory laws and 140 years to achieve equal representation of women in leadership at the workplace [4].

How does this reflect in medicine, notably critical care and perioperative medicine?

1.2 Medical Professionals: Critical Care and Perioperative Medicine

As in any professional working environment, it is accepted that gender inequality weakens the healthcare system and delivery of care [5]. A large percentage of women in healthcare encounter bias and harassment, lack of laws and social protection, as well as lower social status and gender pay gap [5]. The increased number of women in medical schools and residency programs does not reflect in an increased number of women leaders. The leaky pipeline, earlier observed in STEM (science, technology, engineering, and mathematics), also declared in medicine, is a metaphorical reference to the decrease in the number of women at every stage of the career progression [6]. Despite many medical students being women, they remain underrepresented in leadership roles and decision-making positions. This has an impact on their career advancement, progression within hierarchies, opportunities for authorship in research publications, appointments as editors or board members of scientific journals, presidency of scientific societies, speakers at conferences, and leadership positions in guideline committees [6–8].

This is more pronounced in some specialities compared to others: critical care medicine and anaesthesia (general acute and surgery disciplines) are among those most affected by women's underrepresentation and gender pay gap [9].

In a recently performed study that explored perceived drivers (or influencing factors) and implications (associated consequences) of gender inequity in critical care medicine, both women and men participants described as prevalent implications the following [10]:

- Women in critical care medicine do not feel respected, valued, or secure in their work. They need to prove their worth constantly and experience both subtle and overt discrimination.
- Lack of diversity in decision-making influences the development and future of the speciality.

Women recognize critical care medicine as a dominantly men environment with the tendency to exclude women and other minorities. On the other hand, men tend to believe that women inherently dislike high-pressure medical specialties [10]. However, there is no inherent reason why women should avoid positions of authority or strain. Recent surveys of anaesthesia professionals have shown that both women and men equally aspire to leadership roles but face similar obstacles, which seem to affect women more [11–13]. One of the most prominent and most difficult to overcome is childbearing, which places a woman in the position of increased strain of work and challenged work-life balance. The idea that all women prioritize work-life balance over ambition and career goals is a myth. Both men and women cite increased workload and working hours as obstacles to pursuing leadership positions, as these factors reduce time available for family, friends, or personal time [11]. To add, data on LGBT+ population are lacking.

Although macro inequities could be easy to recognize as obvious discrimination, they are rarely seen nowadays. A culture of gender bias and inequality has generated microinequities that are subtle, frequently transient, hidden, hard to prove, and difficult to identify [14]. For example, in one Swedish study it has been shown that to have a comparable score on grant applications, women researchers need to have three times more first authorships, have 2.5 times more publications, or publish in journals with a higher impact factor [1, 15]. The use of the h-index to assess scientists' contributions has become increasingly common in many scientific fields and this also applies in medicine and STEM. This metric is used in departments and universities to make important decisions about hiring, promotions, raises, and awards. A growing body of research shows that there are gender differences in citations and h indices. To illustrate the importance of this effect, the observed gender effect was translated into a meaningful metric—that of salary—and showed that the gender difference in the h index could translate into significant financial costs for female faculty [16].

An additional bonus to known microinequities is that women are less likely to be introduced as doctors during the rounds [17].

Still, there is a research gap in this area of gender equality. Many studies that analyse disaggregated data are from high-income countries, have methodological flaws and tend to focus solely on the numbers and structures of women's underrepresentation [5]. There are many open questions regarding the reasons behind the present disparities and the most effective ways to address them. We still have lack of knowledge what is happening in low- and middle-income countries with the data of workforce structure missing.

It has been recognized that the system needs changes, but somehow it is always expected that women will lean in, meaning that they should adjust and overcome with their efforts the existing frame of inequity [18].

1.3 Patients and Healthcare Systems

In terms of health, equality of conditions refers to the ability of men and women to realize their full rights and potential for health, to contribute to the advancement of health, and benefit from the results. Healthcare professionals strive to deliver safe, patient-centred, efficient, and equitable care. Sex and gender differences impact the full spectrum of critical care medicine, from critical care access to the severity of presentation, initial and ongoing management, and to short- and long-term outcomes. Despite significant advancements in critical care medicine, limited attention has been given to sex and gender disparities in management and outcomes of patients admitted to the intensive care unit (ICU). While "sex" pertains to biological and physiological characteristics, such as reproductive organs, chromosomes and sex hormones, "gender" refers more to sociocultural roles and human behaviour. Unfortunately, data on gender-related topics in the ICU are lacking [19]. Although the lack of equal representation of women professionals in leadership and decision-making positions is disturbing and challenging, of considerable concern are inequities in access to the healthcare system and different outcomes that may depend on disparities in medical care.

During the 1990s, in cardiovascular medicine, several landmark studies have proven the first inequalities in medical care [20]. It was revealed that women often received different treatment in acute coronary care setting compared to men, which was associated with worse outcomes. Within the years, it became clear that aside from bias, research has widely disregarded sex and gender differences, with women being regularly underrepresented in clinical trials and experimental research, affecting the usual clinical practice [20]. There could be an unfortunate interplay between disparities of care based on gender bias and discrimination, or different access to the healthcare system from one side, and genuine sex and gender differences on the other, that alter the course of illness, diagnosis, clinical care, and outcomes.

Today, in critical care medicine, biological factors (sex) and sociocultural factors (gender) are recognized as factors of influence in different manners which are explored in other chapters.

Outcomes after critical illness, often referred to as the post-intensive care syndrome (PICS), encompass a range of issues, some of which are associated with sex differences in frequency and presentation [21]. ICU-acquired weakness is detected in long-stay ICU patients and female sex has consistently been identified as an independent risk factor in multiple international studies and meta-analyses [22]. While the underlying mechanism remains unclear, this diagnosis significantly impacts women's ability to regain functional independence, manage care transitions, return to work, and reintegrate into the community [23].

Biological differences in sex hormone profiles and immune responses seem to modify the trajectory of critical illness in common ICU diagnoses like sepsis or ARDS [20]. However, evidence remains equivocal at this time, given the underrepresentation of women and the lack of information regarding hormonal status, hormone intake, and cyclic changes in many studies. Undertreatment remains not to be limited to these diagnoses and affects the general female population, starting from less-frequent ICU admissions to less organ support measures—despite being equally ill [20]. The underlying reasons for these inequalities remain unclear, but unconscious or implicit bias may influence the treating clinicians, leading to delays in diagnosis and care with harmful consequences. The implementation of validated gender scores and the Sex and Gender Equity in Research (SAGER) in critical care research may help to detangle the impact of biological and gender factors on critical illness [24].

Anaesthesiology professionals have been pioneering safe medicine and are leaders in efforts to obtaining patient safety and professional well-being. Despite that, it has been recognized that infant or maternal mortality, unmanaged acute and chronic pain are disproportionately prevalent in patients that may be subjected to bias and discrimination [25].

One of the examples is racial and ethnic disparities in the rates of neuraxial anaesthesia for caesarean delivery in the USA, where general anaesthesia is used almost double for black women compared to non-Hispanic White women (11.3% versus 5.2%) [26]. The reasons are not yet well understood, but they may arise from the patient (health literacy, understanding of their medical conditions, treatment choices, trust in the healthcare system), provider (unconscious bias, communication barriers), or healthcare system (hospital resources, insurance policies) [25]. This pattern of practice is of particular concern regarding safety because neuraxial anaesthesia is generally offering several advantages for both mother and child.

Also, a greater socio-economic disadvantage is leading to reduced access to epidural anaesthesia during labour, explaining how intersectionality contributes to disparities in women's health. This pattern persists even among women with a medical indication for epidural analgesia and is more pronounced in non-white ethnicities [27]. Data indicates that increasing socio-economic disadvantage may be associated with a range of adverse maternal characteristics, such as maternal BMI, comorbidities, smoking, and illicit drug use, which can contribute to adverse perinatal outcomes [27]. Women from different socio-economic backgrounds and levels of education may lack knowledge about the indications for epidural analgesia, face life circumstances that adversely impact antenatal care attendance, mistrust medical staff, feel disempowered during labour, hold misconceptions about the safety of epidural analgesia, or have different expectations and societal pressures regarding the pain of childbirth [27].

Sex- and gender-informed medicine is another, new paradigm of clinical practice and medical research that considers the association of sex and gender with each element of the disease process from risk to presentation, and to response to therapy [28]. Still, many gaps in knowledge remain. A culture of change and provision of better healthcare will only be realized when perspectives of the differences in sex and gender become incorporated in educational curricula from medical schools throughout ongoing professional development.

1.4 Where Do We Go from Here?

Undoubtedly, there are many reasons to address gender equality, equity, diversity, and inclusion in society and medicine. Projected lack in the workforce, challenges, and crises in public health as Covid-19 pandemic was [29], great public expectations, patient-centred care, and individualized medicine, as well as future technology and scientific expansion, need to have all individuals involved in their full abilities and potential. Still, we have many active participants left behind.

Very often, gender equality, equity, diversity, and inclusion are in the focus, without much progress. We face a diverse world, with countries that have cultural, religious, social, and economic differences, creating everyday challenges in politics and disturbing environmental changes. Healthcare professionals may have a diversity of professional interests and advancement towards education, research, or a variety of subspecialties, but fairness and equal opportunities should be a common goal and interest for all of us.

In this opening chapter, we lay the groundwork for a critical examination of diversity, equality, equity, and inclusion or the current lack of them, in perioperative and critical care medicine. As we explore the complexities of this issue, we invite our readers on an enlightening journey to understand and challenge the status quo.

Join us in this pivotal endeavour, as we confront biases, celebrate diversity, and build bridges towards excellence in our fields. Our collective efforts will not only enhance the quality of care for our patients but also foster a work culture where every member can thrive. Together, we will champion a brighter, more compassionate future for all who touch and are touched by perioperative and critical care medicine.

References

1. Neskovic V. What we talk about when we talk about gender equality and equity in anaesthesia and intensive care. Editorial E-MJA. 2023;7(3):9–12. https://doi.org/10.55302/MJA237304n.
2. https://www.youtube.com/watch?v=-DW4HLgYPlA. Kimberlé Crenshaw - On intersectionality – keynote – WOW 2016.

3. https://sdgs.un.org/goals#history
4. https://sdgs.un.org/goals/goal5
5. Delivered by women, led by men: a gender and equity analysis of the global health and social workforce. Geneva: World Health Organization.; 2019 (Human Resources for Health Observer Series No. 24). Licence: CC BY-NC-SA 3.0 IGO.
6. Bosco L, Lorello GR, Flexman AM, Hastie MJ. Women in anaesthesia: a scoping review. Br J Anaesth. 2020;124(3):e134–47. https://doi.org/10.1016/j.bja.2019.12.021.
7. Flexman AM, Shillcutt SK, Davies S, Lorello GR. Current status and solutions for gender equity in anaesthesia research. Anaesthesia. 2021;76(Suppl 4):32–8. https://doi.org/10.1111/anae.15361.
8. Rubulotta F, Mehta S, Parson LJ. Intensive care medicine: reflections on the gender gap. ICU Management & Practice. 2020;20(4):319–24.
9. https://assets.publishing.service.gov.uk/media/5fd893a7e90e076631fb2286/Gender_pay_gap_in_medicine_review.pdf
10. Leigh JP, Grood C, Ahmed SB, et al. Toward gender equity in critical care medicine: a qualitative study of perceived drivers, implications, and strategies. Crit Care Med. 2019;47(4):e286–91. https://doi.org/10.1097/CCM.0000000000003625.
11. Matot I, De Hert S, Cohen B, Koch T. Women anaesthesiologists' attitudes and reported barriers to career advancement in anaesthesia: a survey of the European Society of Anaesthesiology. Br J Anaesth. 2020;124(3):e171–7. https://doi.org/10.1016/j.bja.2020.01.005.
12. Zdravkovic M, Osinova D, Brull SJ, et al. Perceptions of gender equity in departmental leadership, research opportunities, and clinical work attitudes: an international survey of 11 781 anaesthesiologists. Br J Anaesth. 2020;124(3):e160–70. https://doi.org/10.1016/j.bja.2019.12.022.
13. Zdravkovic M, Neskovic V, Berger-Estilita. J surveys on gender issues among anaesthesiologists: where do we go from here? J Gend Stud. 2021;30(7):868–71. https://doi.org/10.1080/09589236.2021.1969225.
14. Rowe M. Micro-affirmations & Micro-inequities. J Int Ombudsman Assoc. 2008;1:45–8.
15. Noronha B, Fuchs A, Zdravković M, Berger-Estilita J. Gender balance in the medical workplace—a snapshot into anesthesia. Trends Anaesth Crit Care. 2022;43:4–10. https://doi.org/10.1016/j.tacc.2022.02.004.
16. https://sfdora.org/
17. Files JA, Mayer AP, Ko MG, et al. Speaker introductions at internal medicine grand rounds: forms of address reveal gender bias. J Womens Health (Larchmt). 2017;26:413–9.
18. Ryan M. To advance equality for women, use the evidence. Nature. 2022;604(7906):403. https://doi.org/10.1038/d41586-022-01045-y.
19. Lat TI, McGraw MK, White HD. Gender differences in critical illness and critical care research. Clin Chest Med. 2021;42(3):543–55. https://doi.org/10.1016/j.ccm.2021.04.012.
20. Merdji H, Long MT, Ostermann M, et al. Sex and gender differences in intensive care medicine. Intensive Care Med. 2023;49(10):1155–67. https://doi.org/10.1007/s00134-023-0719.
21. Herridge MS, Azoulay É. Outcomes after critical illness. N Engl J Med. 2023;388(10):913–24. https://doi.org/10.1056/NEJMra2104669.
22. De Jonghe B, Sharshar T, Lefaucheur JP, et al. Paresis acquired in the intensive care unit: a prospective multicenter study. JAMA. 2002;288(22):2859–67. https://doi.org/10.1001/jama.288.22.2859.
23. Pandharipande PP, Girard TD, Jackson JC, et al. Long-term cognitive impairment after critical illness. N Engl J Med. 2013;369(14):1306–16. https://doi.org/10.1056/NEJMoa1301372.
24. Heidari S, Babor TF, De Castro P, Tort S, Curno M. Sex and gender equity in research: rationale for the SAGER guidelines and recommended use. Res Integr Peer Rev. 2016;1:2. Published 2016 May 3. https://doi.org/10.1186/s41073-016-0007-6.
25. Toledo P, Adams J. Why a focus on diversity, equity, and inclusion is a perioperative patient quality and safety imperative. APSF Newslett. 2022;37(43):45–6.
26. Toledo P, Eosakul ST, Grobman WA, et al. Primary spoken language and neuraxial labor analgesia use among hispanic medicaid recipients. Anesth Analg. 2016;122:204–9.

27. Halliday L, Shaw M, Kyzayeva A, Lawlor DA, Nelson SM, Kearns RJ. Socio-economic disadvantage and utilisation of labour epidural analgesia in Scotland: a population-based study†. Anaesthesia. Published online February 15. 2024;79:473. https://doi.org/10.1111/anae.16236.
28. Bartz D, Chitnis T, Kaiser UB, et al. Clinical advances in sex- and gender-informed medicine to improve the health of all: a review. JAMA Intern Med. 2020;180(4):574–83. https://doi.org/10.1001/jamainternmed.2019.7194.
29. Myatra S, Rubulotta F. Working in the pandemic and preserving diversity. ICU Manag Pract. 2021;21(4):182–4.

How to Read This Book: Key Features for Fostering Diversity and Well-Being in Perioperative and Critical Care Medicine

2

Francesca Rubulotta and Vojislava Neskovic

2.1 Introduction

This book offers a ground-breaking holistic approach to addressing the gender gaps in perioperative and critical care medicine, emphasizing the association between gender medicine, patient outcomes, and healthcare provider well-being. Before starting to read and use the information and knowledge from this book, we as the editors would like to point out the advantages, unique features, and practical guidance on how to read it.

2.2 Unique Features: Holistic Approach

While numerous reviews, data, and reports highlight the gaps in perioperative and critical care medicine, this book takes an innovative approach not only identifying the source of the problem but also proposing comprehensive solutions which will be called "action plans". The editors and authors of this book have a commendable and forward-thinking approach that recognizes the interconnectedness of patients' safety with the providers' well-being. This perspective is vital in promoting what is

F. Rubulotta (✉)
Department of Anaesthesia and Critical Care, Ospedale Gaspare Rodolico Catania, Catania, Italy

International Women in Intensive and Critical Care Medicine, iWIN ETS, Catania, Italy
e-mail: francesca.rubulotta@unict.it

V. Neskovic
Clinic for Anesthesia and Critical Care, Faculty of Medicine MMA, Military Medical Academy, Belgrade, Serbia

V. Neskovic, F. Rubulotta (eds.), *Diversity, Gender Equity and Inclusion in Critical Care and Perioperative Medicine*,
https://doi.org/10.1007/978-3-031-86286-1_2

defined as the "holistic approach" to the future of perioperative and critical care medicine.

This book encloses some unique features:

- Offers evidence-based strategies and interventions for promoting diversity, equity, and inclusion (DEI) in perioperative and critical care medicine.
- Provides theoretical concepts, practical guidance, and real-world examples to help healthcare professionals and organizations implement DEI initiatives effectively.
- Highlights the importance of supporting healthcare providers in promoting DEI.
- Addresses the concept of intersectionality, recognizing that individuals may experience multiple forms of discrimination or disadvantage simultaneously.
- Emphasizes the importance of equity in healthcare delivery, ensuring that all patients receive the care they need regardless of their background or identity.
- Recognizes that improving diversity and inclusion in healthcare settings leads to better patient outcomes. This may include increased patient satisfaction, better adherence to treatment plans, and reduced health disparities among marginalized populations.
- The book may offer strategies for self-care and resilience-building among healthcare professionals and networking. This book includes the need for role models (women, Health in Lesbian, Gay, Bisexual, and Transgender LGBT+, minorities).
- This volume is a testament to the dire need to address burnout, especially amongst women and minorities at the frontline.

DEI in perioperative and critical care medicine and is essential not only for eliminating health disparities but also for optimizing resource allocation, shaping clinical trial design, enhancing patient satisfaction, and promoting the well-being of healthcare providers. The pivotal role that these concepts play in enhancing patient care will unravel throughout the chapters of this unique book as will the numerous practical strategies to address the glaring gaps in representation among genders and minorities in the field. By confronting these issues head-on, this book serves as a foundational text for those eager to engage with these nuanced topics in perioperative and critical care medicine. Falling under the same umbrella of attention, diversity encapsulates the acknowledgment and inclusivity of differences within a setting. In the context of healthcare, diversity spans across a wide array of dimensions including, but not limited to, age, religion, socioeconomic status, abilities, and ethnicity.

2.3 Practical Guidance the Structure of This Book

This book is divided into two parts: the first focuses on patients and the second on healthcare providers.

Part I is dedicated to the principles of DEI as the inseparable part of the patient-centered care system. This segment referring to patients encompasses topics including the positive impact of diversity on patient care and satisfaction, the influence of social biases on treatment, potential discrimination or disparity of care, and the effect of culture and society on patient outcome. Emphasis is put on women's health and patient satisfaction as the important and often neglected outcome. The importance of DEI in healthcare delivery is evaluated ensuring that all patients receive the care they need regardless of their background or identity. The first part addresses the concept of intersectionality, recognizing that individuals may experience multiple forms of discrimination or disadvantage simultaneously. Authors offer various methods to identify discriminatory behaviors and modify the culture.

Part II describes in detail the concept of the gender gap: discussing theoretical concepts, practical guidance, and real-world examples to help healthcare professionals and organizations implement DEI initiatives effectively. Here the role of healthcare professionals, providing essential context, definitions, and indicators are presented. Gender equity, as well as DEI, is an indispensable element in comprehensive healthcare, and refers to fairness in the recognition, distribution, and accessibility of opportunities, resources, and rewards between women, LGBT+, and men, taking into consideration their different needs and potential. Endowed with differing skills and experiences, genders can contribute to enriching the scientific discourse and clinical practice. The book critically evaluates the representation gap of gender and minorities in perioperative and critical care medicine. It analyses global scenarios and actions currently being taken, laying out essential, recommended, and optional changes that can foster a more inclusive working environment.

Targeting healthcare professionals this book is organized in a manner that intends to shed light upon the current challenges while acting as a manual for adopting more equitable and diverse practices. Recognizing the emotional labor involved in addressing sensitive issues related to diversity and inclusion, the book may offer strategies for self-care and resilience-building among healthcare professionals. This section includes the need for role models and networking. The community is crucial, sponsorship combined with efficient mentorship could be the game changer.

In this part, topics were explored in the light of equality and equity.

2.4 Practical Guidance

This international effort is to create awareness and to inspire actions that can tangibly drive positive changes.

Every chapter starts with a short title followed by the abstract. There are keywords and 3 key points from the Editors in each chapter. The text continues with the presentation of 3 objectives which indicate skills and knowledge that will be acquired by reading the chapter. The content of the chapter is divided by some highlights namely: reflection points and boxes. The chapter is completed by a series of tangible action plans, seen as the achievable priorities from the Editors. Those are derived from real-life examples, suggested solutions, and written as expert opinion.

The editors intended to create a book structure that enables interaction and open communication with the readers, encouraging reflection on their own experiences, challenging their attitudes and current knowledge, and hopefully driving change. Reflection points are mostly written as questions to inquire attitudes and personal experience, while boxes contain parts of the authors' text that convey a clear message.

The content covered in this volume is comprehensively tailored to meet the understanding of readers ranging from junior to senior staff members.

While it may also be insightful for patients and their families, guided reading is suggested to prevent potential misunderstandings.

As we cross this fundamental steppingstone of defining these concepts, we embark on a monumental journey to resort to gender equity and diversity as the new prescriptions for excellence in the realms of perioperative medicine and critical, ensuring the resurrection of a resilient and inclusive healthcare infrastructure.

2.5 Reflection Point from the Editors Before You Continue

At the end of this introductory chapters, the editors wish to quote a classic novel by Italian Sicilian playwright Luigi Pirandello: Uno, Nessuno, Centomila (One, No One, and One Hundred Thousand). In this novel, the main character Mr. Moscarda through one small physical flow of his nose realizes that people see him from one thousand nonreconcilable perspectives. This becomes a motive for him to search his true self. This is the story and philosophical experiment on struggle of a man to defending the integrity of his selfhood during the industrial revolution in the face of unjustifiable partialities imposed by society and unconscious biases. While during the industrial revolution people had to integrate in the industrial world, perform like a machine, and dramatically change priorities and lifestyle, in the twenty-first century the public witnesses a new silent revolution. Pirandello's nineteenth century Europe was marked by the establishment of new life rhythms, priorities, and requests which were the result of the industrial revolution and the need to work simulating and as efficiently as machines.

Today, female, LGBT+ , minorities, healthcare providers, researchers, patients and patients representatives witness myriad challenges while their presence is increasing rapidly in perioperative and critical care medicine. Authors have addressed possible risks and immediate challenges to create a productive work environment. *Uno, nessuno and centomila* issues must be recognized and solved. It represents the rational for the book.

Part II

Patients and Families: Introducing Patient-Centred Care to Gender Equity and Diversity

3 Clinical Trials in the Light of Diversity, Gender Equity, and Inclusion. New Funding Policies

María Cruz Martín Delgado, Judith Gutiérrez Gutiérrez, and Antonio Artigas

Key Points from the Editors

- Diversity in clinical trials is essential for ensuring equitable benefits, addressing health disparities, and advancing precision medicine for better outcomes. Lack of diversity leads to non-generalizable scientific evidence.
- Improving representation requires funding research, building infrastructure, supporting education, and raising awareness. Dedicated funding is key to creating an inclusive structure.
- Several policies have been created to increase diversity in clinical trials, focusing on including groups that have been historically underrepresented. While there's no one-size-fits-all solution, it is important to address each barrier to ensure broader participation.

M. C. M. Delgado (✉) · J. G. Gutiérrez
Intensive Care Unit, Hospital Universitario 12 Octubre, Madrid, Spain
e-mail: judit.gutierrez@salud.madrid.org

A. Artigas
Intensive Care Department, Corporacion Sanitaria Universitaria Parc Tauli. Institut d'Investigació i Innovació Parc Tauli (I3PT). Autonomous University of Barcelona, Sabadell, Spain
e-mail: aartigas@tauli.cat

V. Neskovic, F. Rubulotta (eds.), *Diversity, Gender Equity and Inclusion in Critical Care and Perioperative Medicine*,
https://doi.org/10.1007/978-3-031-86286-1_3

Main Objectives
After reading this chapter, you will be able to:

- Support greater diversity in clinical trials by including marginalized groups to ensure research reflects all genetic, cultural, and socio-economic factors, improving treatment effectiveness and equity.
- Identify and address barriers to underrepresentation in clinical trials, such as language, trust issues, limited access, strict eligibility, and logistical challenges, while emphasizing the need for funding and community involvement.
- Describe policies that improve diversity, equity, and inclusion in clinical trials through financial incentives, broader eligibility, community recruitment, education, and the use of technology and AI.

3.1 Introduction: Terminology

Health is a combination of physical and mental well-being, influenced by behaviour, biology, environment, social policies, and life experiences. Personal experiences vary significantly across race and ethnicity, socio-economic status, geographic location, sexual orientation, gender identity, and other socio-demographic characteristics [1].

The goal of clinical research is to enhance the health and well-being of society. Mirroring the triple aim of healthcare, the triple aim for clinical research focuses on improving individual participant's experiences, promoting population health, and reducing the per capita costs of research [2].

People can experience the same disease in different ways. It is crucial that clinical trials incorporate diversity to ensure that all communities benefit from scientific advancements. Health disparities remain a persistent social issue, and the lack of diversity and representativeness in research contributes to non-generalizable evidence, leading to suboptimal health outcomes at the individual level. Beyond improving health equity, representativeness is vital in advancing precision or personalized medicine, ultimately leading to the best possible outcomes for all individuals [3, 4].

Participation in clinical trials should, therefore, reflect those affected by the disease or condition for which the intervention or product is intended. In cases where appropriate epidemiological data is lacking, trial participation should broadly represent the general population while also protecting vulnerable groups [5].

In recent years, the landscape of clinical trials has been evolving, with increasing attention to gender equity and diversity. Historically, clinical trials have been criticized for underrepresenting women, children and minority groups, which has resulted in biases in medical research, drug development, and treatment, limiting biological understanding and perpetuating health inequities and social injustice. New funding policies and regulations are being implemented to address these imbalances, ensuring that clinical trials are more representative of the population [6].

Assessing the representation of different populations in clinical trials, as well as tracking trends over time, is challenging due to the scarcity of data [7]. To enhance transparency in demographic participation, the U.S. Food and Drug Administration (FDA) publishes the *Drug Trials Snapshots* annually. These reports provide data on participants involved in trials that led to FDA approval of new drugs, specifically new molecular entities and biologics [5].

Progress has been made in some areas, particularly in the representation of white women in clinical trials, where over 50% female participation has been achieved in the United States. However, the same progress has not been seen among racial and ethnic minority populations. Additionally, other groups, such as older adults, pregnant and breastfeeding women, LGBTQIA+[1] individuals, and people with disabilities, continue to be underrepresented or even excluded from clinical trials and research [8].

In the field of intensive care medicine, a recent study analysed data from 24 trials with 68,968 participants in total with 36.3% of women included (ranging from 16.6% to 47.8%). Each trial recorded sex, but not gender. The pooled study population has substantially fewer women than the general ICU patient population, suggesting a relative male predominance in the ICU patient groups by design [9].

Health Equity (WHO Definition) [10]:

- The absence of unfair, avoidable, or remediable health differences among population groups, defined by social, economic, demographic, or geographical factors, or other dimensions of inequality (e.g., sex, gender, ethnicity, disability, sexual orientation).
- Achieved when all people can reach their full potential for health and well-being.
- Despite this goal, health systems often fail to meet basic principles of equity.

Gender is a social construct and refers to societal tasks, roles, and characteristics assigned to men and women, whereas sex is assigned at birth and refers to the underlying biological aspects of being male or female [10].

Diversity, equity, and inclusion (DEI) describes policies, programs, and guidelines that encourage the representation and participation of specific populations of people in relation to gender, sex, sexual orientation, race, ethnicity, age, disability, nationality, religion, socio-economic status, culture, and political perspective [11].

Diversity involves all the way that people are different, including the various traits and characteristics that distinguish one demographic or individual from another, inclusion refers to the behaviours and practices that ensure those individuals and groups are valued, permitting diversity to flourish; equitable policies strive

[1] LGBTQIA+ is used as an inclusive term for the various gender identities and sexual orientations, including lesbian, gay, bisexual, transgender, questioning, queer, intersex, asexual, and pansexual.

to ensure that all individuals have equal access to the same opportunities, regardless of background or identity [12].

3.2 Why Diversity in Clinical Research Matters?

Marginalized racial and ethnic groups, women, and other historically underrepresented populations remain significantly excluded from clinical trials, despite growing concern among policymakers, patient advocates, and some industry leaders. The primary goals of increasing diversity in clinical trial participation include building trust, promoting equity, and advancing biomedical knowledge [13].

Historically, clinical trials often failed to recruit participants who accurately represented those most affected by specific diseases, conditions, or behaviours. These trials frequently relied almost exclusively on white male participants, creating significant gaps in understanding disease mechanisms, preventive factors, and treatment efficacy across different populations. Such knowledge gaps can undermine healthcare decision-making, impede risk reduction strategies, compromise treatment effectiveness, and limit the development of more efficacious drugs or interventions [3].

The lack of diversity in clinical trials jeopardizes the generalizability, quality, and external validity of medical research. In many cases, representation cannot be adequately assessed because critical personal characteristics, such as race and gender identity, are inconsistently collected or reported [14].

Biological differences between men and women (gender differences), such as hormonal variations, metabolism rates, and disease prevalence, mean that treatments can have different effects based on sex [15]. But these biological differences do not explain most of the differences found between both genders. Similarly, genetic, cultural, and socio-economic factors can influence health outcomes and treatment responses across ethnic groups [16–18]. The failure to include racially and ethnically diverse populations in clinical trials results in treatments that may be less effective, or could present unknown side effects, for certain groups.

Without adequate diversity in clinical trials, ensuring the efficacy and safety of treatments for different demographic groups—who may respond differently due to genetic, cultural, or environmental factors—is impossible. To ensure that all individuals benefit from medical advancements, it is essential that clinical research includes a broad spectrum of participants.

A report from the National Academies of Science, Engineering, and Medicine (NASEM) on improving representation in clinical trials highlighted the significant costs and consequences of the lack of diversity and representativeness in the US population. Key findings include: [17]

- **Compromised generalizability of clinical research findings**: The scientific evidence generated in clinical trials cannot always be extrapolated to non-represented populations. These groups may exhibit distinct disease presentations or health profiles that affect their responses to investigational drugs or therapies.

Inconsistent therapeutic responses can lead to healthcare delivery that is not evidence-based and may slow innovation and discovery.

- **Substantial financial and social costs**: This lack of representation is reflected in reduced life expectancy, lower rates of disability-free living, and decreased workforce participation, with costs running into the hundreds of billions of dollars.
- **Enhanced recruitment challenges**: Engaging underrepresented populations could alleviate one of the main obstacles in clinical trials—difficulty in recruiting participants—which is often a key factor in trial discontinuation.
- **Restricted access to effective treatments**: When certain populations are excluded from clinical trials, it limits the ability to set evidence-based treatment indications and affects reimbursement decisions for certain therapies.
- **Erosion of trust**: The continued exclusion of marginalized populations from clinical research undermines trust in both the clinical research process and the medical establishment, exacerbating existing health disparities.

3.3 Barriers to Diversity in Clinical Research

Numerous barriers contribute to the underrepresentation of certain stakeholders in clinical trials, ranging from study design to publication in medical journals. A rapid review of the literature conducted by Bodicoat et al [18] identified several key barriers, including language and communication challenges, a lack of trust, limited access to trials, stringent eligibility criteria, attitudes and beliefs, insufficient knowledge about clinical trials, and logistical and practical issues.

The inability or difficulty to read or write in English is one of the most important barriers for some populations in clinical trials in Europe and the United States [19]. Moreover, language barriers also impact individuals with low literacy levels or disabilities.

A pervasive lack of trust in research, healthcare providers, investigators, medications, and the medical industry is another substantial barrier. This mistrust often stems from past negative experiences or serious adverse events reported in studies [20] which can be exacerbated by related beliefs and fears.

Reflection Point How has the COVID-19 pandemic highlighted the impact of mistrust in research and vaccines, particularly among marginalized communities, and what steps can be taken to promote diversity, equity, and inclusion in research to rebuild trust and ensure more equitable health outcomes?

Limited access to clinical trials, due to various reasons, and excessively strict eligibility criteria (inclusion/exclusion criteria) are major obstacles that disproportionately exclude underserved groups. These groups include older adults, pregnant women, individuals with obesity, those with existing or multiple chronic conditions, and persons with severe mental illnesses or diminished capacity to provide consent [21]. Other constraining factors may include requirements for health insurance coverage, internet access, or specific personal information, as well as inflexible trial designs and the necessity for frequent in-person visits and centralized data collection, often without consideration for decentralized or digital alternatives [22].

Personal and familial attitudes and beliefs can also hinder representativeness in clinical trials. Factors such as a lack of personal or family history of the condition under study, stigma associated with the condition, concerns about side effects or the implications of participating in experimental treatments, religious beliefs, perceptions of being treated as a "Guinea pig," feelings of discomfort or lack of respect, privacy concerns, and negative attitudes towards clinical trials all contribute to this barrier [19].

Logistical and practical challenges may also contribute, including a lack of transportation, time constraints related to participation, additional visits or tests, financial burdens associated with participation, childcare and eldercare responsibilities, and potential job loss due to participation, or insurance requirements [23].

Finally, incorporating diversity into clinical trials may incur higher costs, as it often necessitates more complex study designs, larger sample sizes, and additional outreach efforts to recruit a diverse participant pool. However, emerging funding policies aim to mitigate these costs by providing financial incentives for researchers who prioritize diversity in their studies [24].

Facilitators of Successful Inclusion in Clinical Research

The NASEM report identifies several key facilitators essential for achieving inclusivity in clinical trials:[1]

1. Starting with intention and agency to achieve representativeness.
2. Establishing a foundation of trust with participants and the community at large.
3. Anticipating and removing barriers to study participation.
4. Adopting a flexible approach to recruitment and data collection. Implement flexible recruitment strategies and data collection methods, adapting to the needs of diverse participants is critical for enhancing enrolment and retention.
5. Building a robust network by identifying all relevant stakeholders.
6. Navigating scientific, professional peer, and societal expectations.
7. Optimizing the study team to ensure alignment with research goals.
8. Attaining resources and support to achieve representativeness. The investment of time and money are necessary to successfully engage in the long-term strategies and relationship building needed to drive inclusion in studies.

In summary, efforts to enhance representation must include providing financial resources for research teams, establishing long-term community-based infrastructure, offering material and social support for advocates and community organizations, and educating scientists, community members, and relevant stakeholders, as well as potential study participants and their caregivers, about the importance of these efforts. Dedicated funding is essential to build a robust structure that achieves representation by including and engaging all stakeholders.

To improve representation, it is essential to fund research teams, develop community infrastructure, support advocates and organizations, and raise awareness among all stakeholders about the importance of these efforts. Dedicated funding is key to building a structure that engages everyone involved.

3.4 Policies to Improve Research Diversity

Several policies have been developed to enhance diversity in clinical trials, emphasizing the inclusion of historically underrepresented population groups. While no single solution will be definitive, addressing each barrier is essential. A multiplicity of inclusive efforts is required, with all stakeholders in the clinical research enterprise bearing responsibility and accountability for their actions [25].

The NASEM report urges federal agencies, academic institutions, institutional review boards, and the pharmaceutical industry to improve representation and enhance transparency and accountability. It recommends that journal editors, publishers, and the International Committee on Medical Journal Editors consider the representativeness of trials and populations in any publication submissions [18].

A practical guide from the perspective of a trial sponsor that aims to incorporate DEI principles into clinical trials has recently been published. The goal of this guidance is to help ensure that populations who may ultimately benefit from new therapeutic interventions are represented in clinical trial throughout the clinical trial life cycle from the early stages of drug development through approval and commercialization [26, 27].

Numerous toolkits are available to assist trial teams in integrating equity, diversity, and inclusion into their research programs [28]. However, subsequent evaluations suggest that these efforts have had limited effectiveness. The reasons for the insufficient real-world of these well-intentioned commitments remain unclear. This highlights the need for implementation science, an approach focused on understanding why and how interventions, such as diversity commitments, succeed or fail in specific settings [29].

Key Policies Include:

Financial Incentives for Inclusion of Diverse Groups: Tying funding to the inclusion of diverse participants is one of the most effective policies. Funding agencies require detailed plans outlining how underrepresented groups will be recruited. Researchers who fail to comply risk losing funding or facing restrictions [30].

Participant-centric protocols: Study protocols must account for the health literacy levels of participants, their families, and caregivers. Researching and incorporating language commonly used by the general population into participant-facing materials can facilitate comprehension [31].

Demographic distribution: The demographic composition of clinical trial participants should reflect real-world patient populations [32] Collaborating with organizations like the National Minority Quality Forum can assist trial sponsors in setting appropriate demographic targets. For all demographic categories of interest, subgroup analyses should be planned within the protocol and statistical analysis plan to ensure that enrolment targets are met, and statistical methodologies support the validity of these analyses.

Broadening Inclusion Criteria: Historically, clinical trial exclusion criteria have been excessively stringent, leading to the exclusion of many groups. Modern policies advocate for broader inclusion criteria, permitting participation from individuals with comorbidities or traditionally excluded populations, such as older adults, pregnant women, or individuals with disabilities. Representing real-world populations in clinical trials may require the broadening of trial eligibility criteria such as comorbidities, protocol-prohibited medications, and abnormal laboratory test result [33].

Community-Based Recruitment and Participatory Approaches: Strategies that involve communities in the design and development of clinical trials are being implemented to enhance diversity. These policies encourage collaboration with community leaders, non-profit organizations, and local networks to build trust and facilitate access to clinical trials in underserved communities [34].

Education and Awareness Campaigns: Implementing educational initiatives that inform underrepresented communities about the importance of clinical trial participation is vital. A lack of participation often arises from insufficient information or distrust of the medical system.

Monitoring and Auditing Diversity: Establishing monitoring and auditing systems is crucial to ensuring compliance with diversity requirements in clinical trials. Regulatory and funding agencies can mandate regular reports on participant demographics and subgroup outcomes [35].

Compensation: Providing compensation to clinical trial participants and addressing logistical barriers, such as transportation and childcare, can significantly enhance diversity in research. Economic barriers, like the inability to afford time off work or childcare, often prevent individuals from marginalized communities from participating. By offering financial support, these obstacles can be mitigated, making it easier for a broader range of people to take part in trials [36, 37].

Logistical Support: Logistical barriers, such as the need for frequent in-person visits, can also discourage participation, particularly for those with inflexible work or family obligations. Fairness requires that these logistical challenges be addressed, for example, by offering transportation assistance or flexible scheduling. Efforts must also ensure that the burdens of participation are shared equitably across all groups who stand to benefit from a study's results, avoiding the overburdening of any one community [36, 37].

Digitalization and Technology: Digitizing clinical study procedures can reduce access barriers and lessen the burden of participation. The *e-consent* enables personalized information in the patients' and family environments [37]. Digital tools facilitate remote visits and data collection for patients with geographic, resources or time constraints [38, 39].

Artificial Intelligence (AI): AI has the potential to transform clinical trials by enhancing diversity and representativeness, ultimately leading to more equitable healthcare outcomes. AI can improve participant recruitment, refine trial design, and ensure bias-free data analysis, making clinical trials more inclusive. However, careful consideration must be given to algorithmic biases, ethical concerns, and the need for transparent, inclusive data practices. With appropriate safeguards, AI can help ensure clinical trials reflect the populations they intend to serve. Although several barriers need to be addressed it will be essential to begin with representative patient population models and to connect existing and future artificial intelligence–based recruitment methods with real-world outreach and recruitment strategies that are proven effective [39].

Reflection Point Money serves different purposes in compensation versus logistical support. Compensation directly addresses the economic burden of participation by reimbursing participants for their time, lost wages, or effort. It ensures that individuals, especially from lower-income backgrounds, are fairly compensated for their involvement in the study.

In contrast, logistical support uses money to remove practical barriers, such as covering transportation or childcare costs. This helps participants overcome obstacles that might otherwise prevent them from joining, without directly compensating for their time. Together, both types of support make clinical trials more accessible and equitable for diverse populations.

3.5 Regulatory Requirements Related to Diversity in Clinical Research

To support gender equity and diversity in clinical trials, funding bodies and regulatory agencies are updating their requirements. These policies aim to ensure that research is inclusive and that trial outcomes are relevant to the broader population. These policies provide clear guidelines on how evidence-generating tools (such as new technologies or methods) should be used to improve access to clinical trials, particularly for diverse groups of people. The goal is to make clinical trials more accessible by decentralizing the process—i.e., by allowing trials to take place outside traditional settings like academic medical centres. This could involve things like remote monitoring, virtual visits, or community-based recruitment, which help to involve a wider range of participants, especially those who might otherwise have difficulty accessing trials.

Agencies such as the National Institutes of Health (NIH), the U.S. FDA and other international bodies have introduced policies that directly link funding to the inclusion of women and minorities in clinical trials.

NIH's Inclusion Across the Lifespan and Gender Policy*:* Since 1993, the NIH has required the inclusion of women and minorities in all clinical research it funds [40, 41], In 2019, the NIH expanded this policy to encompass participants across all age groups, including older adults and all genders, unless a scientific justification for exclusion is provided. This policy is significant as it ties compliance directly to funding, meaning that researchers who fail to prioritize diversity risk losing financial support. Research proposals must now include a section detailing how women, minorities, and individuals across the lifespan will be included in the study, along with justifications for any exclusions.

In 2016, the ***FDA released guidance*** requiring companies to report demographic subgroup data (gender, race, and age) in clinical trials [41]. This policy ensures the collection, analysis, and reporting of gender-specific data, allowing for a targeted evaluation of treatment effects. Drug trials seeking FDA approval must now include subgroup analyses to assess whether different genders or ethnicities respond differently to treatments, ensuring that drugs are evaluated not only on average populations but also for specific demographic groups.

US Food and Drug Omnibus Reform Act (FDORA) 2022 Sponsors must submit "diversity action plans" to the FDA for certain late-stage trials, including all Phase 3 trials, unless waived or excepted. These plans should include the following: Goals for enrolment in the clinical study; Rationale for the above goals; and Explanation of how the goals will be met [42].

Horizon Europe sets [43] gender equality as a cross-cutting principle and aims to eliminate gender inequality and intersecting socio-economic inequalities throughout research and innovation systems, including by addressing unconscious bias and systemic structural barriers. The strengthened provisions for gender equality under Horizon Europe address three different levels and include the following [44]:

- A new eligibility criterion to get access to Horizon Europe funding: public bodies, research organizations and higher education establishments from Member States and Associated Countries are required, as of calls with deadlines in 2022, to have in place a gender equality plan (GEP).
- The integration of the gender dimension into research and innovation content across the Program is an operational objective for Horizon Europe and becomes **a requirement by default.**
- Ensuring gender balance, with a target of 50% women in Horizon Europe-related advisory bodies such as boards and expert groups, as well as in evaluation panels. Gender balance among researchers involved in projects is strongly encouraged as well and will be considered as a ranking criterion for ex aequo proposals.

Organizations such as the European Medicines Agency (EMA) and other global entities are adopting similar frameworks, leading to a global push for diversity in medical research.

These regulatory changes have fundamentally transformed clinical trial conduct, making diversity and gender equity prerequisites for financial support. Key impacts of these new policies include:

(a) **Enhanced Study Designs**:
  - Requirement for gender-specific analysis: Funding agencies now mandate researchers to structure their clinical trials in a way that allows for gender-specific data analysis. This means that trial results must be stratified by gender, ensuring that any gender-based differences in treatment outcomes or side effects are identified.
  - Inclusion of diverse populations: Trials are now designed to actively recruit from racially and ethnically diverse populations. This is increasingly seen as not just a regulatory necessity, but a scientific one, as companies and researchers recognize that genetic, environmental, and cultural factors affect health outcomes.

(b) **Increased Funding for Studies Focusing on Underrepresented Groups:** To promote inclusivity, many funding bodies are offering additional grants and incentives for studies that prioritize gender equity and diversity.
  - NIH's Specialized Centres of Research Excellence (SCORE) program supports interdisciplinary research focusing on women's health and gender-based analysis [45].
  - The Patient-Cantered Outcomes Research Institute (PCORI) provides grants specifically targeting research on underrepresented populations, particularly women and minorities [46].
  - Some countries offer tax incentives or government subsidies for companies developing treatments for conditions disproportionately affecting women or minorities.

(c) **Market Access and Drug Development**: For pharmaceutical companies, funding policies linked to diversity are critical as they influence market access. Many drug approvals—particularly in the United States, EU, and increasingly in China—require diversity and subgroup analysis in clinical trials to ensure drug effectiveness across different populations.

Question of Reporting in Research

- Researchers almost two decades ago highlighted the need for reporting the primary outcome of trials disaggregated by sex or gender to provide more equitable and inclusive evidence [47].
- The Sex and Gender Equity in Research (SAGER) guidelines, published in 2016, aim to standardize sex and gender reporting in research [48].
- There is no significant improvement in ex and gender-based analysis (SGBA) reporting or female participant inclusion, with cardiology trials showing better SGBA than ICU trials.
- Acute care trial participants are mostly white, and fewer than 30% of trials report race or ethnicity; demographic factors like income or education are rarely included.
- The reasons for the lack of progress in SGBA reporting, despite the SAGER guidelines, remain unclear.

The White House Initiative on Women's Health Research is a comprehensive effort to spur innovation in women's health and ensure federally funded research benefits everyone [49].

Funding bodies and research institutions increasingly focus on community engagement strategies and culturally tailored recruitment approaches. NIH and FDA guidelines encourage researchers to work with community leaders and local organizations to build trust and ensure that recruitment is done ethically and inclusively. Finally, funding agencies are providing additional resources for recruitment, retention, and analysis of diverse populations to alleviate the financial burden of meeting diversity mandates.

3.6 Conclusion

The research community has an imperative to make DEI principles key foundational aspects in study conduct to pursue better personalized medicine for diverse patient populations. Clinical research should be conducted in representative study samples to generate evidence that can guide practice with greater confidence in predictable outcomes and safety profiles in different populations.

Improving representation in clinical research requires a substantial investment of time, money, and effort. Also, improving representation requires transparency and accountability and must be present at all points in the research life cycle.

Clinical research involves multiple stakeholders (participants, communities, investigators, IRBs, industry sponsors, institutions, funders, regulators, journals, and policymakers). Each of them has a critical role to play in achieving the goal of improving representation in clinical research.

Proposed Actions

- Address the limited impact of current equity, diversity, and inclusion toolkits, further research on identifying key barriers and enablers, empowering trial teams to refine strategies for more effective and sustainable integration of diversity and equity should be encouraged. This action will improve understanding why efforts in existing recommendations and strategies succeed or fail in practice.
- Enhance enforcement by journal editors and peer reviewers to promote sex- and gender-based analysis (SGBA) in clinical trials. Address concerns about subgroup testing and sex-specific disease prevalence, while prioritizing improved diversity reporting and female participant recruitment in acute care trials. Ensure the implementation of the SAGER Guidelines.
- Horizon Europe promotes gender equality as a cross-cutting principle, aiming to eliminate gender and socio-economic inequalities in research and innovation, addressing unconscious bias and systemic barriers.

- New eligibility criterion: Public bodies, research organizations, and higher education institutions must have a gender equality plan (GEP) to access funding, starting from calls in 2022.
- Integrating gender into research and innovation content is a key operational objective and a requirement under Horizon Europe.
- Gender balance is targeted at 50% women in advisory bodies, boards, expert groups, and evaluation panels, with gender balance in project teams also considered in proposal rankings.

References

1. Diversity and Inclusion in Clinical Trials. https://www.nimhd.nih.gov/resources/understanding-health-disparities/diversity-and-inclusion-in-clinical-trials.html#resources. [Accessed 04 September 2024].
2. Dorsey ER, Kieburtz K. The triple aim of clinical research. Clin Trials. 2021;18(4):511–3. https://doi.org/10.1177/17407745211001522. Epub 2021 Apr 20. PMID: 33878933; PMCID: PMC8292156
3. Washington V, Franklin JB, Huang ES, Mega JL, Abernethy AP. Diversity, equity, and inclusion in clinical research: a path toward precision health for everyone. Clin Pharmacol Ther. 2023;113(3):575–84. https://doi.org/10.1002/cpt.2804. Epub 2022 Dec 15. PMID: 36423203
4. Cwalina TB, Jella TK, Manyak GA, Kuo A, Kamath AF. Is our science representative? A systematic review of racial and ethnic diversity in orthopaedic clinical trials from 2000 to 2020. Clin Orthop Relat Res. 2022;480(5):848–58. https://doi.org/10.1097/CORR.0000000000002050. Epub 2021 Dec 2. PMID: 34855650; PMCID: PMC9007212
5. Bierer BE, Meloney LG, Ahmed HR, White SA. Advancing the inclusion of underrepresented women in clinical research. Cell Rep Med. 2022;3(4):100553. https://doi.org/10.1016/j.xcrm.2022.100553. PMID: 35492242; PMCID: PMC9043984
6. National Academies of Sciences, Engineering, and Medicine; Policy and Global Affairs; Committee on Women in Science, Engineering, and Medicine; Committee on Improving the Representation of Women and Underrepresented Minorities in Clinical Trials and Research; Bibbins-Domingo K, Helman A, editors. Improving Representation in Clinical Trials and Research: Building Research Equity for Women and Underrepresented Groups. Washington (DC): National Academies Press (US); 2022 May 17. 3, Policies to Improve Clinical Trial and Research Diversity: History and Future Directions. Available from: https://www.ncbi.nlm.nih.gov/books/NBK584404/ [Accessed 04 September 2024].
7. Alegria M, Sud S, Steinberg BE, Gai N, Siddiqui A. Reporting of participant race, sex, and socioeconomic status in randomized clinical trials in general medical journals, 2015 vs 2019. JAMA Netw Open. 2021;4(5):e2111516. https://doi.org/10.1001/jamanetworkopen.2021.11516. PMID: 34037736; PMCID: PMC8155820
8. National Academies of Sciences, Engineering, and Medicine; Policy and Global Affairs; Committee on Women in Science, Engineering, and Medicine; Committee on Improving the Representation of Women and Underrepresented Minorities in Clinical Trials and Research; Bibbins-Domingo K, Helman A, editors. Improving Representation in Clinical Trials and Research: Building Research Equity for Women and Underrepresented Groups. Washington (DC): National Academies Press (US); 2022 May 17. Summary. Available from: https://www.ncbi.nlm.nih.gov/books/NBK584393/ [Accessed 04 September 2024].
9. Modra L, Bone A, Pilcher D, Woodward M, Thompson K. Sex representation within intensive care trials in Australia and New Zealand. Intensive Care Med. 2024;50(9):1529–31.

https://doi.org/10.1007/s00134-024-07541-1. Epub 2024 Jul 16. PMID: 39012536; PMCID: PMC11377652

10. van Diemen J, Verdonk P, Chieffo A, Regar E, Mauri F, Kunadian V, Sharma G, Mehran R, Appelman Y. The importance of achieving sex- and gender-based equity in clinical trials: a call to action. Eur Heart J. 2021 ;42(31):2990–2994. doi: https://doi.org/10.1093/eurheartj/ehab457. Erratum in: Eur Heart J 2021 Oct 14;42(39):4048. https://doi.org/10.1093/eurheartj/ehab583. PMID: 34352884; PMCID: PMC8370758.
11. Gichane MW, Griesemer I, Cubanski L, Egbuogu B, McInnes DK, Garvin LA. Increasing diversity, equity, and inclusion in the health and health services research workforce: a systematic scoping review. J Gen Intern Med. 2024; https://doi.org/10.1007/s11606-024-09041-w. Epub ahead of print. PMID: 39320587
12. Servaes S, Choudhury P, Parikh AK. What is diversity? Pediatr Radiol. 2022;52(9):1708–10. https://doi.org/10.1007/s00247-022-05356-0. Epub 2022 Mar 29. PMID: 35348810; PMCID: PMC8962281
13. Schwartz AL, Alsan M, Morris AA, Halpern SD. Why diverse clinical trial participation matters. N Engl J Med. 2023;388(14):1252–4. https://doi.org/10.1056/NEJMp2215609. Epub 2023 Apr 1. PMID: 37017480
14. Carter-Edwards L, Hidalgo B, Lewis-Hall F, Nguyen T, Rutter J. Diversity, equity, inclusion, and access are necessary for clinical trial site readiness. J Clin Transl Sci. 2023;7(1):e268. https://doi.org/10.1017/cts.2023.660. PMID: 38380391; PMCID: PMC10877510
15. Ivan S, Daniela O, Jaroslava BD. Sex differences matter: males and females are equal but not the same. Physiol Behav. 2023;259:114038. https://doi.org/10.1016/j.physbeh.2022.114038. Epub 2022 Nov 22. PMID: 36423797
16. Zucker I, Prendergast BJ. Sex differences in pharmacokinetics. Handb Exp Pharmacol. 2023;282:25–39. https://doi.org/10.1007/164_2023_669. PMID: 37439843
17. National Academies of sciences, engineering, and medicine. Improving representation in clinical trials and research: building research equity for women and underrepresented groups. Washington, DC: National Academies Press, 2022.
18. Bodicoat DH, Routen AC, Willis A, Ekezie W, Gillies C, Lawson C, Yates T, Zaccardi F, Davies MJ, Khunti K. Promoting inclusion in clinical trials-a rapid review of the literature and recommendations for action. Trials. 2021;22(1):880. https://doi.org/10.1186/s13063-021-05849-7. PMID: 34863265; PMCID: PMC8643184
19. Byrne MM, Tannenbaum SL, Glück S, Hurley J, Antoni M. Participation in cancer clinical trials: why are patients not participating? Med Decis Mak. 2014;34(1):116–26. https://doi.org/10.1177/0272989X13497264.
20. Lee GE, Ow M, Lie D, Dent R. Barriers and facilitators for clinical trial participation among diverse Asian patients with breast cancer: a qualitative study. BMC Womens Health. 2016;16(1):43. https://doi.org/10.1186/s12905-016-0319-1. Accessed 06 Oct 2024
21. Shepherd V, Wood F, Griffith R, Sheehan M, Hood K. Protection by exclusion? The (lack of) inclusion of adults who lack capacity to consent to research in clinical trials in the UK. Trials. 2020;19:474.
22. Dulko D, Kwong M, Palm ME, Trinquart L, Selker HP. From a decentralized clinical trial to a decentralized and clinical-trial-in-a-box platform: towards patient-centric and equitable trials. J Clin Transl Sci. 2023;7(1):e236. https://doi.org/10.1017/cts.2023.629. PMID: 38028335; PMCID: PMC10663768
23. Williams CP, Deng L, Caston NE, Gallagher K, Angove R, Pisu M, Azuero A, Arend R, Rocque GB. Understanding the financial cost of cancer clinical trial participation. Cancer Med. 2024;13(8):e7185. https://doi.org/10.1002/cam4.7185. PMID: 38629264; PMCID: PMC11022148
24. Igwe JK, Wangdak Yuthok TY, Cruz E, Mueller A, Lan RH, Brown-Johnson C, Idris M, Rodriguez F, Clark K, Palaniappan L, Echols M, Wang P, Onwuanyi A, Pemu P, Lewis EF. Opportunities to increase science of diversity and inclusion in clinical trials: equity and a lack of a control. J Am Heart Assoc. 2023;12(24):e030042. https://doi.org/10.1161/JAHA.123.030042. Epub 2023 Dec 18. PMID: 38108253; PMCID: PMC10863780

25. Kelsey MD, Patrick-Lake B, Abdulai R, Broedl UC, Brown A, Cohn E, Curtis LH, Komelasky C, Mbagwu M, Mensah GA, Mentz RJ, Nyaku A, Omokaro SO, Sewards J, Whitlock K, Zhang X, Bloomfield GS. Inclusion and diversity in clinical trials: actionable steps to drive lasting change. Contemp Clin Trials. 2022;116:106740. https://doi.org/10.1016/j.cct.2022.106740. Epub 2022 Mar 29. PMID: 35364292; PMCID: PMC9133187
26. Versavel S, Subasinghe A, Johnson K, Golonski N, Muhlhausen J, Perry P, Sanchez R. Diversity, equity, and inclusion in clinical trials: a practical guide from the perspective of a trial sponsor. Contemp Clin Trials. 2023;126:107092. https://doi.org/10.1016/j.cct.2023.107092. Epub 2023 Jan 23. PMID: 36702295
27. US Food and Drug Administration, Enhancing the Diversity of Clinical Trial Populations — _Eligibility Criteria, Enrollment Practices, and Trial Designs Guidance for Industry. https://www.fda.gov/regulatory-information/search-fda-guidance-documents/enhancing-diversity-clinical-trial-populations-eligibility-criteria-enrollment-practices-and-trial, 2020, 2020. Accessed 4 Oct 2024.
28. Kuaban A, Force ASoCTaHET. ASH DEI Toolkit for Clinical Trial Sponsors: Incorporating DEI Principles throughout the Clinical Collister D, et al. BMJMED 2024;3:e000984. doi:https://doi.org/10.1136/bmjmed-2024-000984 3 Trial Life Cycle. American Society for Hematology, 2023. Available: https://www.hematology.org/-/media/hematology/files/dei/ashdei-toolkit-for-clinical-trial-sponsors.pdf.
29. Collister D, Song C, Ruzycki SM. Fostering diversity in clinical trials: need for evidence and implementation to improve representation. BMJ Med. 2024;3(1):e000984. https://doi.org/10.1136/bmjmed-2024-000984. PMID: 39175921; PMCID: PMC11340663
30. Clark SG, Cohen A, Heard-Garris N. Moving Beyond Words: Leveraging Financial Resources to Improve Diversity, Equity, and Inclusion in Academic Medical Centers. J Clin Psychol Med Settings. 2023 Jun;30(2):281–287. doi: https://doi.org/10.1007/s10880-022-09914-4. Epub 2022 Dec 10. PMID: 36495346; PMCID: PMC9739343.
31. Arumugam A, Phillips LR, Moore A, Kumaran SD, Sampath KK, Migliorini F, Maffulli N, Ranganadhababu BN, Hegazy F, Botto-van BA. Patient and public involvement in research: a review of practical resources for young investigators. BMC Rheumatol. 2023;7(1):2. https://doi.org/10.1186/s41927-023-00327-w. PMID: 36895053; PMCID: PMC9996937
32. Gomez LE, Bernet P. Diversity improves performance and outcomes. J Natl Med Assoc. 2019;111(4):383–92. https://doi.org/10.1016/j.jnma.2019.01.006. Epub 2019 Feb 11. PMID: 30765101
33. Not-PatientSpecific-Solutions. 2021. Accessed 25 October 2022. [27] D.C. St Germain, W. McCaskill-Stevens, Use of a clinical trial screening tool to enhance patient accrual, Cancer. 127 (10) (2021) 1630–1637.
34. Milton AJ, Flores EJ, Charles EF, Elezaby MA, Ward EC, Lee CI, Woods RW, Martin Rother MD, Strigel RM, Narayan AK. Community-based participatory research: a practical guide for radiologists. Radiographics. 2023;43(5):e220145. https://doi.org/10.1148/rg.220145. PMID: 37104126; PMCID: PMC10190132
35. Corsino L, Fuller AT. Educating for diversity, equity, and inclusion: a review of commonly used educational approaches. J Clin Transl Sci. 2021;5(1):e169. https://doi.org/10.1017/cts.2021.834. PMID: 34733545; PMCID: PMC8532179
36. Chatters R, Dimairo M, Cooper C, Ditta S, Woodward J, Biggs K, Ogunleye D, Thistlethwaite F, Yap C, Rothman A. Exploring the barriers to, and importance of, participant diversity in early-phase clinical trials: an interview-based qualitative study of professionals and patient and public representatives. BMJ Open. 2024;14(3):e075547. https://doi.org/10.1136/bmjopen-2023-075547. PMID: 38508621; PMCID: PMC10952868
37. Skelton E, Drey N, Rutherford M, Ayers S, Malamateniou C. Electronic consenting for conducting research remotely: a review of current practice and key recommendations for using e-consenting. Int J Med Inform. 2020 Nov;143:104271. https://doi.org/10.1016/j.ijmedinf.2020.104271. Epub 2020 Sep 13. PMID: 32979650; PMCID: PMC7487205.
38. Coran P, Goldsack JC, Grandinetti CA, Bakker JP, Bolognese M, Dorsey ER, Vasisht K, Amdur A, Dell C, Helfgott J, Kirchoff M, Miller CJ, Narayan A, Patel D, Peterson B,

Ramirez E, Schiller D, Switzer T, Wing L, Forrest A, Doherty A. Advancing the use of Mobile Technologies in Clinical Trials: recommendations from the clinical trials transformation initiative. Digit Biomark. 2019;3(3):145–54. https://doi.org/10.1159/000503957. PMID: 32095773; PMCID: PMC7011727

39. Askin S, Burkhalter D, Calado G, El Dakrouni S. Artificial intelligence applied to clinical trials: opportunities and challenges. Health Technol (Berl). 2023;13(2):203–13. https://doi.org/10.1007/s12553-023-00738-2. Epub 2023 Feb 28. PMID: 36923325; PMCID: PMC9974218
40. Bernard MA, Clayton JA, Lauer MS. Inclusion across the lifespan: NIH policy for clinical research. JAMA. 2018;320(15):1535–6. https://doi.org/10.1001/jama.2018.12368. PMID: 30326521
41. US Food and Drug Administration, US Department of Health and Human Services. Diversity plans to improve enrollment of participants from underrepresented racial and ethnic populations in clinical trials: guidance for industry. Draft guidance. Available: https://www.fda.gov/media/157635/download [Accessed 06 October 2024].
42. Peloquin D, Barnes M, Lam C. Congress enacts legislation requiring guidance on clinical research diversity and modernization. Ropes & Gray. Available: https://www.ropesgray.com/en/insights/alerts/2023/01/congress-enacts-legislation-requiring-guidance-on-clinicalresearch-diversity-and-modernization [Accessed 06 October 2024].
43. Gender equality in research and innovation https://research-and-innovation.ec.europa.eu/strategy/strategy-2020-2024/democracy-and-rights/gender-equality-research-and-innovation_en [Accessed 06 October 2024].
44. Cederroth CR, Earp BD, Gómez Prada HC, Jarach CM, Lir SA, Norris CM, Pilote L, Raparelli V, Rochon P, Sahraoui N, Simmon C, Vissandjee B, Mour C, Arbogast M, Armengol JM, Mason R. Integrating gender analysis into research: reflections from the gender-net plus workshop. EClinicalMedicine. 2024;13(74):102728. https://doi.org/10.1016/j.eclinm.2024.102728. PMID: 39105192; PMCID: PMC11299571
45. Specialized Centers of Research Excellence on Sex Differences (U54 Clinical Trial Optional). https://orwh.od.nih.gov/sex-gender/orwh-mission-area-sex-gender-in-research/specialized-centers-of-research-excellence-on-sex-differences-u54-clinical-trial#:~:text=The%20Specialized%20Centers%20of%20Research,on%20the%20health%20of%20women.
46. Fischer MA, Asch SM. The future of the Patient-Centered Outcomes Research Institute (PCORI). J Gen Intern Med. 2019;34(11):2291–2. https://doi.org/10.1007/s11606-019-05324-9. PMID: 31529376; PMCID: PMC6848293
47. Granton D, Rodrigues M, Raparelli V, et al. Sex and gender-based analysis and diversity metric reporting in acute care trials published in high-impact journals: a systematic review. BMJ Open. 2024;14:e081118. https://doi.org/10.1136/bmjopen-2023-081118.
48. Heidari S, Babor TF, De Castro P, et al. Sex and gender equity in research: rationale for the SAGER guidelines and recommended use. Res Integr Peer Rev. 2016;1:2.
49. Mazure CM. The white house initiative on women's health research. JAMA Intern Med. 2024; https://doi.org/10.1001/jamainternmed.2024.3592. Epub ahead of print. PMID: 39348106

4 Global Health and Women: Looking Beyond Maternal Health

Sheila Nainan Myatra, Gauri Raman Gangakhedkar, and Sukhada Savarkar

Key Points from the Editors

- Discriminatory attitudes among healthcare providers, resulting from insufficient training on women's health needs, lead to delays in diagnosis and lower standards of care. These disparities are more pronounced in resource-limited countries.
- While maternal health is crucial, women's longer lifespans involve chronic conditions that impact their roles as caregivers and society members. Focusing on reproduction overlooks women without children or diverse sexual orientations. There is an increasing need to broaden the focus to women's health since non-communicable diseases are the leading causes of death among women.
- Overcoming barriers for women in global health requires training, creating supportive environments, and adapting systems to local needs, while increasing female leadership to reduce biases and promote equality in healthcare.

S. N. Myatra (✉) · G. R. Gangakhedkar · S. Savarkar
Department of Anesthesiology, Critical Care and Pain, Tata Memorial Hospital, Homi Bhabha National Institute, Mumbai, India

V. Neskovic, F. Rubulotta (eds.), *Diversity, Gender Equity and Inclusion in Critical Care and Perioperative Medicine*,
https://doi.org/10.1007/978-3-031-86286-1_4

Main Objectives

After reading this chapter, you will be able to:

- Analyse the priorities within healthcare systems regarding women's maternal and non-maternal health.
- Explain the impact of non-communicable diseases on global women's health.
- Identify the factors—such as bias, gender-based stereotypes and inequities, lack of knowledge, socioeconomic status, and differences in funding and policymakers between countries—that affect global women's health.

4.1 Introduction

Women play central roles in family and community wellbeing, healthcare provision, and substantial—albeit under recognized—contributions to economic development. In many low- and middle-income countries (LMICs), with increasing urbanization and changes in family structure, women have been taking on more responsibility as breadwinners while maintaining traditional household and caregiving responsibilities.

Globally, roles and opportunities are determined by socially and culturally accepted gender norms, which have an impact on social and structural factors which in turn influence health, health risk habits, as well as the availability and acceptable standard of healthcare and social services. It has long been understood that gender-related barriers and inequalities influence women's access to health care and available health resources.

As a result, though women generally have greater healthcare needs over their life course, they often have fewer resources and less autonomy to access or pay for healthcare, even if services are free or subsidized [1, 2]. These challenges are often amplified, on account of lower literacy rates, racial, socio-economic, age-based or sexual-orientation-based marginalization, leading to disparities that span over generations.

Thus, ending discrimination against women and girls is not only a basic human right, but an absolute need of our times. The United Nations has determined "Gender Equality" as the fifth sustainable development goal of 17. They recognize that empowering women and promoting gender equality is crucial to accelerating sustainable development, and also has the potential to have a multiplier effect across other development areas.

4.2 Impact of Gender-Based Health Inequality

Unfortunately, these gender inequalities appear to be embedded in our health systems and reflect as unconscious gender biases based on gender-based stereotypes and sexism [3].

Since men and women have different physiologies, their health needs differ as well. However, women's health has traditionally received less focus as compared to men's health, particularly from an intervention perspective. One of the most important examples of this bias is that most of the basic medical data comes from research that has been acquired from trials which recruited only male participants.

Though it seems like simple logic now that men and women be represented equally in all trials, the FDA and US government only made it mandatory for women to be participants in trials sponsored by the National Institute of Health in 1993 [4]. Historically, the data acquired from women through trials has been famously mired with the injustice inflicted on the unwitting participants, with Henrietta Lacks and acquisition of the HeLa cell line, her family being the most renowned example [5].

The differences in male and female physiologies translate into differences in pharmacokinetics and/or pharmacodynamics for drugs, which could potentially result in differences in safety or efficacy. For example, oestrogen lengthens the cardiac repolarization time, leaving women more vulnerable to the development of Torsade de Pointes arrhythmias on administration of drugs that lead to QT-prolongation (like ondansetron, amiodarone) [6]. Similarly, women also experience 30–40% higher serum concentrations and thus complications with loop diuretics, and are at a higher risk bleeding complications with unfractionated or low molecular weight heparin [7].

These biases persist even in the clinical management of patients arriving at healthcare setups, both in the implicit and the explicit forms. In fact, a large volume of evidence has been accrued in recent years that unequivocally proves, that men and women approaching the healthcare system with similar complaints are treated differently [8, 9]. A landmark paper by Maserejian et al. showed the existence of this disparity when middle-aged men and women complained of chest pain [10]. The physicians were significantly less certain about the aetiology of chest pain in female patients ($p = 0.006$) and female patients were twice as likely to be given a mental health diagnosis as opposed to coronary artery disease as compared to the men. Similar findings were elicited in studies conducted in patients with psoriasis, neck pain and polypharmacy [11].

Women suffering from out-of-hospital cardiac arrests appear to be at a significant disadvantage. They are less likely to present with a shockable rhythm, and a larger proportion of their incidents occur at home and go unwitnessed, compared to men [12, 13]. Social concerns such as allegations of sexual misconduct, as was emphasized by a public survey conducted in the USA induce a sense of reluctance in initiating CPCR [14]. Unfortunately, even achieving return of spontaneous circulation does not equalize their chances of receiving definitive interventions such as targeted temperature management, invasive mechanical circulatory support, percutaneous coronary intervention (PCI), and coronary artery bypass grafting (CABG) [12, 15].

One would presume that once a critically ill patient reaches the intensive care unit (ICU), gender-based differences in treatment would disappear, given that established validated and purely clinical criteria are used to determine the appropriate line of management. However, for most clinical conditions, ICU admissions are provided less frequently to women compared to men, even though large meta-analyses suggest that the severity of illness on ICU admission was found to be either similar or higher in women [16, 17]. For instance, studies on sepsis suggest that 61% of patients with septic shock are men, showing a male preponderance, and the 1-hour sepsis bundle is 38% more likely to be completed, and had received the first dose of antibiotics 34% faster as a median value [18].

A particularly detrimental line of thought is seen to drive these decisions. Women are more frequently seen to set limits to treatment, particularly in higher age groups, leading to a clinician bias where they assume that women beyond a certain age may prefer less aggressive care [19]. This clinical bias can result in catastrophic consequences wherein women are less likely to receive early goal-directed therapies, invasive procedures, and other organ support measures such as mechanical ventilation and renal replacement therapy (RRT) [18, 20].

Our literature search thus leads us to understand that implicit/explicit discriminatory attitudes exist even among healthcare providers; owing to the lack of training and awareness among healthcare providers and health systems to the specific health needs and challenges faced by women contributing to a delay in diagnosis and a delay or even denial of care.

However, stronger advocacy and better representation by international leaders has resulted in increasing attention towards women's health issues. The introduction of Millenium Development Goals (MDG) by the United Nations with the subsequent involvement and support of individual government have led to local initiatives to streamline global health objectives for women. The 2015, "Global Leaders" Meeting on "Gender Equality and Women's Empowerment: A Commitment to Action" hosted by UN General Assembly ensured financial commitments totalling US$25 billion, and garnered substantial political support [21]. Key identifications from this meeting were sex-based health disparities are far greater in resource-limited countries, where women lack basic health care and face debilitating and life-threatening health issues, some of which have been eradicated many years ago in developed countries. As a result, the policies and initiatives formed to accomplish MDGs focus heavily on the issues that plague women in LMICs.

4.3 Current Healthcare Policies for Maternal and Childcare

Women of reproductive age and children form two-thirds of the global population [22]. Annually, 250,000–280,000 women die during pregnancy and childbirth, with most of these deaths during or immediately after childbirth [23]. Of the 6.55 million children under the age of 5 who die annually, 3.5% of them die within the first 28 days of their lives [24]. The numbers suggest that the under-five mortality in LMICs is 56 times more than that in high-income countries (HICs) [24]. Poor maternal health care and nutrition, maternal infections, and other poor conditions contribute to increased maternal and neonatal morbidity and mortality [25].

It is a bald fact that the burden presented by the morbidity and mortality in women in the reproductive age group is simply staggering and most maternal and child deaths are largely preventable. Deaths occur most frequently, through labour, delivery and the immediate post-partum period. Two-thirds of the deaths can be attributed to post-partum haemorrhage, puerperal infections, pregnancy-induced hypertension and complications from unsafe abortions [26]. 80% of the neonatal deaths have aetiologies that can be traced to the peri-partum period [27]. Since 50 million births and 77% of all neonatal deaths occur in places where women do not have access to both ante-natal healthcare and the presence of a Skilled Birth Attendant (SBA) at the time of delivery, simple intervention of introducing universal antenatal care and ensuring the presence of an SBA can prove to be a key solution [28–30]. Furthermore, application of the effective medical know-how required to address both the situations comprises of cheap and easy to implement solutions that would require minimal training of medical and para-medical staff in addition to strengthening the available infrastructure. As a result, policymakers recognize that health interventions targeting this population are likely to have a long-term impact on a nation's economic and social development, which is why much of the growing focus on addressing gender-based inequality in healthcare continues to prioritize maternal health.

Every new-born: an action plan to end preventable deaths (ENAP) and targets and strategies for ***Ending preventable maternal mortality (EPMM)*** represent the multi-agency international roadmap that consists of clear implementable strategies that aim at reducing the global maternal mortality ratio (MMR) to less than 70 per 100,000 live births, neonatal mortality to at least as low as 12 per 1000 live births and under-5 mortality to at least as low as 25 per 1000 live births and 12 or fewer stillbirths per 1000 total births in all countries [31]. The ENAP and EPMM have developed shared targets with these objectives in mind. In collaboration with country governments, the aim is to provide four or more antenatal contacts, presence of SBA during the delivery and provision of early routine post-natal care as critical high-impact basic packages of care.

Reflection Point The preventable morbidity and mortality among women in the reproductive age group, particularly during labour, delivery, and the post-partum period, highlights the urgent need for universal antenatal care and skilled birth attendants. With simple, cost-effective interventions, many lives could be saved, especially in areas lacking access to basic healthcare. How can policymakers accelerate the implementation of these straightforward solutions to improve maternal and neonatal health? What long-term impact could this have on social and economic development?

4.4 Need for Changing Priorities

While the steadily increasing interest in improving maternal health is to be lauded indeed, one must bear in mind that reproductive lifespan forms only a fraction of a woman's life. Currently available data tells us that the average lifespan for women is higher than that for men all around the world (3.82–5.22 years) [32]. However, this belief cannot be generalized, since studies exploring survival after myocardial infarction and stroke have shown ambiguous results [33]. In reality, what longer average lifespans for women tell us is that though women report more illnesses than men, and are more likely to live in poor conditions, they can survive chronic conditions such as stable cardiovascular diseases, cancers, and disabilities for longer than men [33]. Their longer lifespans allow women to contribute to family finances and continue their socially delegated role as caregivers for far longer than their reproductive life span. Focussing solely on maternal and reproductive health also marginalizes and excludes those women who either choose to and are unable to bear children and those with non-heterosexual sexual orientation [30].

Additionally, the global burden of disease among women has changed significantly in the last couple of decades, with non-communicable diseases (NCDs) gradually becoming the leading causes of death and disability for women in almost all countries of the world. In fact, according to WHO global health estimates; 7 out of 10 leading causes of death among women were NCDs in 2019, compared to four out of ten top causes of death in 1990 [34].

This knowledge implores us to improve focus on women's health, particularly conditions which continue to chronically affect women and in turn, their capacity to be caregivers and productive society members.

4.5 Non-communicable Diseases

In recent times, major transitions have occurred in global health such as decline in death rates, increase in life expectancy, ageing of populations, and a dramatic shift from deaths at younger ages, mainly due to infectious diseases, to non-communicable diseases. Data shows that NCDs are responsible for the highest disease burden worldwide. They are dominating mortality figures at a global level not only in men but also in women. Deaths due to NCDs have long since surpassed maternal mortality rates worldwide. Women collectively spend about 20% more years living with disability (YLDs) due to NCDs [34].

Despite this glaring concern of NCDs, the role of NCDs in women's health has been sidelined globally. The current global strategies do not sufficiently address them. For example, over 50% of the health budget allocated by the US Agency for International Development is for reproductive and maternal health [35].

This limitation of women's health to reproductive health is evident in private donations and philanthropic funding as well. Ford Foundation funded 1300 grants for women's health from 1999 through the first quarter of 2004. Out of these 1300 grants; only two were allocated for cancer and none for diabetes or cardiovascular disease [36].

Several assumptions and myths have contributed to the neglect of NCDs in women. The strong historical ties between the concept of women's health and reproductive health are largely responsible for the lack of holistic approach towards women's health [37]. NCDs are responsible for two out of every three deaths among women each year and yet women's health has been defined only through their reproductive capacity [38].

This approach of focusing solely on reproduction and child rearing has been quite aptly termed by Nanette Wenger as the "bikini approach" [39]. It tends to ignore the rest of the woman and health problems that are specific to women but not directly related to reproduction, such as domestic violence. It also ignores health problems that women share with men, like non-communicable disease, cancer, etc.

In addition, historically, NCDs have been considered primarily as diseases of men. Research has now proven that nothing can be further from the truth. Cardiovascular diseases, cancer, and chronic respiratory diseases are the top three causes of death in women globally [30, 40]. In fact, the incidence and severity of some chronic diseases are more in women compared to men owing to biological and other social determinants that affect women disproportionately. For example, around 40% of the world's population and 90% of rural households in LMICs use wood, coal, charcoal, or animal waste for cooking. Women share an unequal burden of cooking responsibilities and spend substantial periods close to these biofuel sources while cooking indoors. This places them at a disproportionately higher risk of developing chronic pulmonary diseases due to exposure to air pollution caused by the burning of biofuels over open fire [41].

Contrary to the belief that NCDs in women are an issue only in high-income countries, data suggests that most of the NCD deaths in women occur in low- and middle-income countries. Literature suggests that 77% of all NCD deaths are from low- and middle-income countries [42].

Another disturbing myth is that NCDs cause deaths only in older people. Unfortunately, a significant proportion of deaths from NCDs in low- and middle-income countries are under the age of 70 years [43]. In the 2014 systematic analysis of the global causes of maternal deaths, maternal deaths were divided into direct (obstetric-related) and indirect causes. Deaths due to NCDs were considered amongst the fraction of "indirect" maternal deaths. The analysis found that indirect causes contributed to significant proportion of (27%) maternal deaths [44].

Therefore, the approach of improving women's health must broaden to include NCDs as they are responsible for the greatest burden of ill health. NCD prevention activities should be incorporated into already existing maternal and women-centric programmes.

4.5.1 Cancer

Despite advances in the understanding and treatment of cancer, cancer is a leading cause of death and disability around the world. In 2020, there were 18.1 million cancer cases globally out of which 8.8 million were women. In 2012, 522,000 and

266,000 women died of breast and cervical cancer respectively which means close to half a million more women died from these two cancers alone than from complications of pregnancy or childbirth [26, 45]. While the maternal mortality rates have reduced significantly over the past three decades; breast cancer incidence and mortality are increasing annually, at a rate of 3.1% and 1.8%, respectively [46]. These statistics emphasize the unmet challenges in cancer care, especially in women.

Furthermore, cancer poses significant public health challenges especially in low- and middle-income countries. It is emblematic of the inequities faced by LMIC where the epidemiological transition is shifting the burden of disease to chronic, non-communicable diseases coupled with an overlapping backlog of illness associated with preventable infections, poverty, and reproductive health problems.

Cancers that primarily affect women present significant challenges in terms of achieving health equity. The incidence and diagnosis of cancer, access to health care and treatment is significantly dependent on where a woman lives, what is the social, financial status of her in society, how early she presents, whether she has access to affordable treatment services. This is strikingly seen for cervical cancer, as around 85% of women diagnosed with cervical cancer and 88% of women who die from cervical cancer live in a LMIC [41]. HPV vaccination is a proven approach to prevent cervical cancer, yet the access and availability to HPV vaccination is limited for most women in many countries with low resources.

On the other hand, breast cancer is the most common cancer among women in almost all countries which includes the high-income as well as low-income countries.

This "double burden" of cervical and breast cancer that is faced by LMIC is characteristic of the cancer transition. Although incidence of cervical cancer is declining in most high-income countries, it is far from controlled in LMICs. Therefore, women in low-resource setting are facing a dual cancer burden which includes potentially preventable cancers and all other cancers for which primary prevention is still difficult with existing scientific knowledge.

A variety of factors like biological, social, environmental and economic factors ultimately lead to gender and sex differences in cancer diagnosis and outcomes [47]. Beyond anatomical and biological factors, gender inequities at individual, relational, and institutional level are responsible for differences in cancer outcome between men and women.

A recent analysis of 128 oncology trials shows that sex and gender terminologies were used inconsistently while reporting the results [48]. None of the studies described how sex and gender information was collected, assessed, or segregated. Without disaggregation of research data by sex and gender, a correct understanding of how sex differences and gender inequalities affect health is not possible. Studies also show that gynaecological cancers are more likely to be underfunded compared with male-dominant other cancers. These disparities in funding and research resources can result in gaps in the evidence-based treatment of female-specific cancers [47]. It can also lead to attrition in the number of researchers who are invested in identifying novel therapies for these diseases.

Huge inequities exist in cancer diagnosis, treatment and survival for women worldwide. Cancer causes a huge economic and emotional burden on women and their families at an individual level. It also causes massive economic burden on national and social economy. Hence urgent international efforts are needed to reduce the cancer burden.

4.5.2 Mental Health

Mental health disorders are major contributors to the global health burden. Recent statistics show that about one in eight people in the world live with a mental disorder [49]. The prevalence of mental disorders also varies with sex. Women are 50% more likely to have mental illness than men. In women, depression alone is responsible for around 41.9% of the disability from neuropsychiatric disorders. Whereas in men, it accounts for 29.3%.

Research shows that men and women respond to stressful triggers differently based on their stereotypical social roles in society and the expectation of behaving in a certain way based on gender [50]. The reason for this difference is multifactorial which includes interaction of physical, reproductive, and biological factors with social, political, and economic and environmental issues. The greater vulnerability of women to mental illness can be due to physiological and genetic changes along with social factors like poverty, sexual abuse, intimate partner violence, the societal expectation from women to bear children, low autonomy in decision-making, and so on.

In majority of cultures worldwide, women play multiple roles such as childbearing and child-rearing, running the family, caring for sick relatives, and earning income which can lead to considerable stress.

Stepanikova et al. did a subgroup analysis of ELSPAC-CZ cohort study which was initiated by the WHO to examine maternal and child health across several European countries [51]. The investigators tried to analyse the perceived gender discrimination that women experience in their everyday life. More than 1 in 10 women—who were either pregnant or parenting young children—said yes for experiencing perceived gender discrimination. They also had higher depression scores than other women. This study emphasizes the role of perceived gender discrimination in a woman's mental health. This subtle form of discrimination is so ingrained in our society that it needs international cooperation from health and social advocates, and from government and policymakers of all genders to reverse it [52].

4.6 Gender-Based Violence

Gender-based violence is an unfortunate pervasive practice that affects 35% of the women globally [53]. Gender-based violence can lead to a large range of physical and mental health problems, which include depression, anxiety, post-traumatic stress disorder, injuries, sexually transmitted infections, unplanned and unwanted pregnancies, and even death [54]. Since such acts of violence are not only a violation of basic rights, but also prevent women from exercising their other social, economic and political rights, they can by no means be deemed acceptable.

Victims of gender-based violence are often subjected to some degree of discrimination by healthcare providers based on the socio-cultural perceptions about gender and their pre-determined roles in society. Unfortunately, this includes stereotypically ascribing certain behaviours to certain genders, for instance aggression among men and subservience among women and a systematic acceptance of gender-based domestic violence. Believing that the victims are responsible for the violence and inadequate training with respect to the handling of victims of gender-based violence cause further damage to their approach towards the victims [54]. These socio-cultural beliefs are deep-rooted and extend even among the victims themselves who often choose to deliberately put the assault behind them to avoid intense scrutiny, judgement and alienation in society, and they may even choose to continue to suffer ongoing abuse rather than report the same to avoid the economic and social ramifications of the same. Since women are taught since a young age that they are the supposedly "weaker" sex, they often believe that they are less capable of standing up or defending themselves [55].

Healthcare systems and healthcare providers are often a first point of call for women and may be the only places where they are allowed visit by themselves. They have a unique vantage point, where they can not only identify the women who are victims of gender-based violence, but also provide a place of trust, to allow disclosure. Empathetic well-trained healthcare providers can help women to access the support they need and potentially help reduce gender-based violence.

The World Health Organization (WHO) **developed guidelines** for the healthcare sector [56]

- Responding to intimate partner violence and sexual violence against women: WHO clinical and policy guidelines (2013).
- Health care for women subjected to intimate partner violence or sexual violence: clinical handbook (2014).

An in-service curriculum based on these documents is designed to equip healthcare providers with the knowledge and skills to implement WHO recommendations in clinical practice.

Training healthcare providers is essential for improving the health system's response to violence against women.

4.7 Women in Healthcare

Women comprise 70% of the healthcare system as frontline health workers and caregivers. However, they fill only 25% of senior and 5% of top positions in healthcare systems, thus forming a minority in global health leadership [57]. As a result, they are often underrepresented when decisions regarding health policy, funding, and research are made.

Women leaders have been known to exhibit more empathy and understanding towards the underprivileged and marginalized populations as is evidenced by their better response to community needs and ensure greater focus on allocation of funds towards education, health, and nutrition, in contrast to their male counterparts [58]. The lack of female representations in the hallowed halls that finally take decisions leads to the exclusion of these invaluable insights.

The ingrained patriarchy and implicit gender biases seep into the lives of the healthcare providers too. Women are usually held to a higher standard for measuring performances, their assertiveness is often perceived as aggression, and are frequently delegated the less recognized tasks [59]. These subtle acts of bias condition the mindset of women in healthcare from the time of their training to such a degree that a study found that women residents expressed higher levels of stress, chose less assertive mannerisms and felt disadvantaged, when thrust in leadership roles [60].

Addressing the barriers that prevent women from breaking the glass ceiling in global health requires training and equipping the women trainee, suitably modifying the work environment to create a more inclusive and supportive work culture and creating processes and organizational systems, that allow adaptation to fit local needs [58]. Increasing the representation of women as leaders in healthcare is a step forward in reducing the biases faced by women in healthcare systems.

"Delivered by Women, Led by Men" the World Health Organization gender and equity analysis of the global health and social workforce (2019) (57)

- Horizontal and vertical gender segregation persist in healthcare, driven by stereotypes.
- Gender discrimination contributes to the underrepresentation of women in leadership positions, with women holding only 25% of leadership roles despite making up 70% of the healthcare workforce.
- Women in healthcare face bias, harassment, lack of legal protections, lower social status, and a gender pay gap.
- Gender inequality is found to weaken the healthcare system and the delivery of care.
- Most of the available data comes from high-income countries, with gaps in research and methodology, limiting the ability to make general conclusions or propose solutions.

4.8 Future Directions

Efforts and initiatives taken by various agencies nationally and internationally have caused significant improvement in maternal mortality. Similar efforts are needed in other aspects of women's health. It is essential that we let go of the traditional bikini approach and embrace a holistic approach to improve women's health.

Thankfully, over the past two decades, global health initiatives have expanded their focus from a narrow emphasis on reproductive health to a broader approach to women's overall health. This expanded "life-course" approach includes health challenges that affect women beyond reproductive years. It also incorporates ailments which they share with men (like NCDs, cancer), perhaps with a greater severity.

Policies and programmes must therefore address women's health from a life-course perspective which focuses on providing women with a continuum of care throughout various phases of life. A strong partnerships and cooperation between governments, the private sector, national and international agencies can go a long way to implement these policies.

Women's contributions to health care by way of taking care of health of their family and community are huge in terms of hours and value. However, significant proportion of these contributions remain unpaid and undervalued [61]. Caregiver-supportive policies must be enforced by government and other civic bodies to value women's contributions as members of the health-care workforce and caregivers.

To take a holistic approach towards women's health, increasing women's education is crucial. Education of women is essential in changing gender norms, to increase awareness about basic human rights as women and to improve their health and their children's health. Government bodies at a local and national level must have gender-responsive education policies that ensures girls' access to quality education and prioritize girls' school attendance to at least secondary school level.

Currently, there are crucial gaps in our understanding of sex and gender differences that can affect the course and outcome of diseases [62]. Therefore, health studies and research projects should disaggregate study data by sex and gender. Recommendations and conclusions made from studies should consider sex and gender differences. Additionally, policies should be developed to include sex and gender systematically into research which will help policymakers to make evidence-based recommendations for improving women's health. Adequate funding should be granted by government agencies and private philanthropy to the studies which are directed towards women's health beyond reproduction.

4.9 Conclusion

Pro-active partnerships with communities, politicians, international organizations, and governments are key to creating deep, transformative changes in women's health. It must be recognized that women's empowerment with regards to health and development is critical to the prosperity of nations. Enhancing women's health is possible only when policies and programmes address women's health holistically and focus on providing women with a continuum of care all through their lives. Shifting away from the narrow view that equates reproductive health with women's overall health is a key aspect of adopting a systems approach to drive this transformation.

Creating these policies would entail taking cognizance of evidence from low- and middle-income countries, thus considering their range of experiences and requirements. These policies, and health systems at large, must address region-specific priorities and challenges while attempting to achieve the global goals. Encouraging and increasing women leaders will help better addressal of gender-specific issues. Above all, women must be encouraged to recognize and speak up about their own healthcare requirements.

"Communities and countries and ultimately the world is only as strong as the health of their women." Michelle Obama.

Proposed Actions

- Raise awareness among the general population, healthcare providers, and policymakers about the importance of prioritizing global women's health, with an emphasis on comprehensive care beyond reproductive health.
- Make education and research on a holistic approach to women's health mandatory in healthcare systems and academic institutions to ensure better understanding and intervention.
- Educate women to challenge and change gender norms, increase awareness of basic human rights, and improve both their own health and the health of their children.
- Educate healthcare professionals on how to manage and care for victims of family or any other form of violence.

References

1. Witter S, Govender V, Ravindran TKS, Yates R. Minding the gaps: health financing, universal health coverage and gender, vol. 32. Oxford University Press; 2017. p. v4.
2. Vijayasingham L, Govender V, Witter S, Remme M. Employment based health financing does not support gender equity in universal health coverage. BMJ. 2020;27(371):m3384.
3. FitzGerald C, Hurst S. Implicit bias in healthcare professionals: a systematic review. BMC Med Ethics. 2017;18(1):19.
4. Liu KA, Mager NA. Women's involvement in clinical trials: historical perspective and future implications. Pharm Pract (Granada). 2016;14(1):708.
5. Baptiste DL, Caviness-Ashe N, Josiah N, Commodore-Mensah Y, Arscott J, Wilson PR, Starks S. Henrietta lacks and America's dark history of research involving African Americans. Nurs Open. 2022;9(5):2236–8.

6. Hammond TG, Valentin JP. Sex differences in ventricular repolarization: from cardiac electrophysiology to Torsades de Pointes. Fundam Clin Pharmacol. 2004;18:139–51.
7. Roosendaal LC, Wiersema AM, Smit JW, Doganer O, Blankensteijn JD, Jongkind V. Editor's choice — sex differences in response to administration of heparin during non-cardiac arterial procedures. Eur J Vasc Endovasc Surg. 2022;64:557–65.
8. Hoffmann D, Tarzian A. The girl who cried pain: a bias against women in the treatment of pain. J Law Med Ethics. 2001;29:13–27.
9. Travis CB, Howerton DM, Szymanski DM. Risk, uncertainty, and gender stereotypes in healthcare decisions. Women Ther. 2012;35:207–20.
10. Maserejian NN, Link CL, Lutfey KL, Marceau LD, McKinlay JB. Disparities in physicians' interpretations of heart disease symptoms by patient gender: results of a video vignette factorial experiment. J Womens Health (Larchmt). 2009;18(10):1661–7.
11. Samulowitz A, Gremyr I, Eriksson E, Hensing G. "Brave men" and "emotional women": a theory-guided literature review on gender bias in health care and gendered norms towards patients with chronic pain. Pain Res Manag. 2018;25(2018):6358624.
12. Lei H, Hu J, Liu L, Xu D. Sex differences in survival after out-of-hospital cardiac arrest: a meta-analysis. Crit Care. 2020;24:613.
13. Lakbar I, Ippolito M, Nassiri A, Delamarre L, Tadger P, Leone M, Einav S. Sex and out-of-hospital cardiac arrest survival: a systematic review. Ann Intensive Care. 2022;12:114.
14. Perman SM, Shelton SK, Knoepke C, Rappaport K, Matlock DD, Adelgais K, Havranek EP, Daugherty SL. Public perceptions on why women receive less bystander cardiopulmonary resuscitation than men in out-of-hospital cardiac arrest. Circulation. 2019;139:1060–8.
15. Vallabhajosyula S, Dunlay SM, Barsness GW, Miller PE, Cheungpasitporn W, Stulak JM, Rihal CS, Holmes DR Jr, Bell MR, Miller VM. Sex disparities in the use and outcomes of temporary mechanical circulatory support for acute myocardial infarction-cardiogenic shock. CJC Open. 2020;2:462–72.
16. Viglianti EM, Yek C, Kadri SS. Understanding sex-based differences in intensive care unit mortality: moving beyond the biology. Am J Respir Crit Care Med. 2022;206(11):1306–8.
17. Modra L, Higgins A, Vithanage R, Abeygunawardana V, Bailey M, Bellomo R. Sex differences in illness severity and mortality among adult intensive care patients: a systematic review and meta-analysis. J Crit Care. 2021;65:116–23.
18. Sunden-Cullberg J, Nilsson A, Inghammar M. Sex-based differences in ED management of critically ill patients with sepsis: a nationwide cohort study. Intensive Care Med. 2020;46(4):727–36.
19. McPherson K, Carlos WG 3rd, Emmett TW, Slaven JE, Torke AM. Limitation of life-sustaining care in the critically ill: a systematic review of the literature. J Hosp Med. 2019;14:303–10.
20. Todorov A, Kaufmann F, Arslani K, et al. Gender differences in the provision of intensive care: a Bayesian approach. Intensive Care Med. 2021;47(5):577–87.
21. United Nations. UN secretary-general announces $25 billion in initial commitments to end preventable deaths of women, children and adolescents by 2030. http://www.un.org/sustainabledevelopment/blog/2015/09/un-secretary-general-announces-25-billion-in-initial-commitments-to-end-preventable-deaths-of-women-children-and-adolescents-by-2030/. Accessed 22 Nov 2023.
22. World Health Organization. trends in maternal mortality: 1990 to 2010. Geneva: Switzerland, World Health Organization; 2012.
23. Lassi ZS, Salam RA, Das JK, Bhutta ZA. Essential interventions for maternal, newborn and child health: background and methodology. Reprod Health. 2014;11(Suppl 1):S1.
24. United Nations Children's Fund: Levels and trends in child mortality 2012: Estimates developed by the UN Inter-agency Group for Child Morality Estimation. 2012, UNICEF, WHO, The World Bank and UN population division.
25. The Partnership for Maternal NCH: A Global Review of the Key Interventions Related to Reproductive, Maternal, Newborn and Child Health (RMNCH).PMNCH 2011. Accessed 5 Sept 2023.

26. Maternal health | UNICEF India [Internet]. UNICEFIndia. 2023 [cited 2023 Dec 18]. Available from: https://www.unicef.org/india/what-we-do/maternal-health
27. Lassi Z, Majeed A, Rashid S, Yakoob M, Bhutta Z. The interconnections between maternal and newborn health—evidence and implications for policy. J Matern Fetal Neonatal Med. 2013;26(S1):3–53.
28. Darmstadt GL, Lee ACC, Cousens S, Sibley L, Bhutta ZA, Donnay F, Osrin D, Bang A, Kumar V, Wall SN. 60 million non-facility births: who can deliver in community settings to reduce intrapartum-related deaths? Int J Gynaecol Obstet. 2009;107:S89–S112.
29. Lawn JE, Kerber K, Enweronu-Laryea C, Cousens S. 3.6 million neonatal deaths- what is progressing and what is not? Semin Perinatol. 2010;34(6):371–86.
30. Myatra SN, Tripathy S, Einav S. Global health inequality and women – beyond maternal health. Anaesthesia. 2021;76(Suppl 4):6–9.
31. Improving maternal and newborn health and survival and reducing stillbirth – Progress report 2023 [Internet]. 2023 [cited 2024 Feb 18]. Available from: https://www.who.int/publications-detail-redirect/9789240073678
32. Baum F, Musolino C, Gesesew HA, Popay J. New perspective on why women live longer than men: an exploration of power, gender, social determinants, and capitals. Int J Environ Res Public Health. 2021;18(2):661.
33. Zarulli V, Barthold Jones JA, Oksuzyan A, Lindahl-Jacobsen R, Christensen K, Vaupel JW. Women live longer than men even during severe famines and epidemics. Proc Natl Acad Sci USA. 2018;115(4):E832–40.
34. Global health estimates: Leading causes of death [Internet]. 2024 [cited 2024 Feb 18]. Available from: https://www.who.int/data/gho/data/themes/mortality-and-global-health-estimates/ghe-leading-causes-of-death
35. Raymond S. Improving people's health background paper: foreign aid in the national interest. Washington, DC: US Agency for International Development; 2002.
36. Raymond SU, Greenberg HM, Leeder SR. Beyond reproduction: women's health in today's developing world. Int J Epidemiol. 2005;34(5):1144–8.
37. Bustreo F, Knaul FM, Bhadelia A, Beard J, Araujo de Carvalho I. Women's health beyond reproduction: meeting the challenges. Bull World Health Organ. 2012;90(7):478–478A.
38. Lozano R, Naghavi M, Foreman K, Lim S, Shibuya K, Aboyans V, et al. Global and regional mortality from 235 causes of death for 20 age groups in 1990 and 2010: a systematic analysis for the global burden of disease study 2010. Lancet. 2012;380:2095–128.
39. Wenger NK. You've come a long way, baby: cardiovascular disease in women, problems and prospects. Circulation. 2004;109:558–60.
40. Institute for Health Metrics and Evaluation. The Global Burden of Disease. 2013. http://vizhub.healthdata.org/gbd-compare/#. Accessed 18 Aug 2023.
41. Ginsburg O, Bray F, Coleman MP, Vanderpuye V, Eniu A, Kotha SR, et al. The global burden of women's cancers: a grand challenge in global health. Lancet. 2017;389(10071):847–60.
42. Non communicable diseases [Internet]. 2024 [cited 2024 Feb 18]. Available from: https://www.who.int/news-room/fact-sheets/detail/noncommunicable-diseases
43. Bonita R, Beaglehole R. Women and NCDs: overcoming the neglect. Glob Health Action. 2014;5(7):23742.
44. Say L, Chou D, Gemmill A, Tunçalp Ö, Moller AB, Daniels J, Gülmezoglu AM, Temmerman M, Alkema L. Global causes of maternal death: a WHO systematic analysis. Lancet Glob Health. 2014;2(6):e323–33.
45. Ferlay J, Soerjomataram I, Dikshit R, et al. Cancer incidence and mortality worldwide: sources, methods and major patterns in GLOBOCAN 2012. Int J Cancer. 2015;136:E359–86.
46. Forouzanfar MH, Foreman KJ, Delossantos AM, Lozano R, Lopez AD, Murray CJL, et al. Breast and cervical cancer in 187 countries between 1980 and 2010: a systematic analysis. Lancet. 2011;378:1461–84.
47. Keenan BP, Barr E, Gleeson E, Greenberg CC, Temkin SM. Structural sexism and cancer care: the effects on the patient and oncologist. Am Soc Clin Oncol Educ Book. 2023;43:e391516.

48. Hall M, Krishnanandan VA, Cheung MC, Coburn NG, Haas B, Chan KKW, Raphael MJ. An evaluation of sex- and gender-based analyses in oncology clinical trials. J Natl Cancer Inst. 2022;114(8):1186–91.
49. Mental disorders [Internet]. 2024 [cited 2024 Feb 18]. Available from: https://www.who.int/news-room/fact-sheets/detail/mental-disorders
50. Yu S. Uncovering the hidden impacts of inequality on mental health: a global study. Transl Psychiatry. 2018;8(1):98.
51. Stepanikova I, Acharya S, Abdalla S, Baker E, Klanova J, Darmstadt GL. Gender discrimination and depressive symptoms among child-bearing women: ELSPAC-CZ cohort study. EClinicalMedicine. 2020;4:100297.
52. Vigod SN, Rochon PA. The impact of gender discrimination on a Woman's Mental Health. EClinicalMedicine. 2020 Mar;19(20):100311.
53. Gender-based violence | UNDP. (n.d.). UNDP. Retrieved July 16, 2020, from https://www.undp.org/content/undp/en/home/2030-agenda-for-sustainable-development/people/gender-equality/gender-based-violence.html
54. Kalra N, Hooker L, Reisenhofer S, Di Tanna GL, García-Moreno C. Training healthcare providers to respond to intimate partner violence against women. Cochrane Database Syst Rev. 2021;5(5):CD012423.
55. Huhtanen, H. Gender Bias in Sexual Assault Response and Investigation. Part 1: Implicit Gender Bias. End Violence Against Women International. [Internet].2024. [cited 2024 Feb 18]. Available from: https://evawintl.org/resource-library/?_sft_resource_author=evawi
56. https://iris.who.int/bitstream/handle/10665/349539/9789240039803-eng.pdf?sequence=1
57. World Health Organization delivered by women, led by men: a gender and equity analysis of the Global Health and Social Workforce. Human resources for health observer series; 24. World Health Organization; 2019. [Internet].2024. [cited 2024 Feb 18]. Available from: https://www.who.int/publications/i/item/9789241515467
58. Batson A, Gupta GR, Barry M. More women must lead in global health: a focus on strategies to empower women leaders and advance gender equality. Ann Glob Health. 2021;87(1):67.
59. Bevan V, Learmonth M. 'I wouldn't say it's sexism, except that… it's all these little subtle things': healthcare scientists' accounts of gender in healthcare science laboratories. Soc Stud Sci. 2013;43(1):136–58.
60. Linden JA, Breaud AH, Mathews J, McCabe KK, Schneider JI, Liu JH, et al. The intersection of gender and resuscitation leadership experience in emergency medicine residents: a qualitative study. AEM Educ Train. 2018;2(2):162–8.
61. Langer A, Meleis A, Knaul FM, Atun R, Aran M, Arreola-Ornelas H, et al. Women and health: the key for sustainable development. Lancet. 2015;386(9999):1165–210.
62. Peters SAE, Woodward M, Jha V, et al. Women's health: a new global agenda. BMJ Glob Health. 2016;1:e000080.

Perioperative Management and Care of Critically Ill Pregnant Patients

5

Emilia Guasch, Nicolas Brogly, Fernando Gilsanz, and Vojislava Neskovic

Key Points from the Editors

- Despite current policies aimed at promoting health equity, significant disparities in maternal healthcare persist. Evidence shows that poor health outcomes during pregnancy and childbirth are often the result of inequitable access to timely and appropriate care.
- The perioperative management and care of critically ill pregnant patients require a multidisciplinary approach that considers the unique physiological changes of pregnancy, the severity of the patient's condition, and the specialized competencies of the healthcare team.
- Low- and middle-income countries (LMICs) face particular challenges in delivering high-quality care to pregnant women. A major barrier to reducing maternal mortality in these regions is addressing the "three delays": in deciding to seek care, in reaching a healthcare facility, and in receiving appropriate care upon arrival at the facility.

E. Guasch (✉)
Anesthesia and Reanimation Department. WFSA obstetric anesthesia subcommittee chair., Hospital Universitario Fundación Jiménez Díaz, Madrid, Spain

N. Brogly
Anesthesia and Reanimation, Hospital Universitario Gregorio Marañón, Madrid, Spain

F. Gilsanz
Real Academia Nacional de Medicina. Universidad Autónoma de Madrid, Facultad de Medicina UAM, Madrid, Spain
e-mail: fgilsanz.hulp@salud.madrid.org

V. Neskovic
Clinic for Anesthesia and Critical Care, Faculty of Medicine MMA, Military Medical Academy, Belgrade, Serbia

V. Neskovic, F. Rubulotta (eds.), *Diversity, Gender Equity and Inclusion in Critical Care and Perioperative Medicine*,
https://doi.org/10.1007/978-3-031-86286-1_5

Main Objectives
After reading this chapter, you will be able to:

- Identify key priorities in the treatment of critically ill pregnant patients and analyse how gender bias in critical care may affect these priorities and patient outcomes.
- Analyse the weaknesses in healthcare systems that hinder access to adequate care for pregnant patients, particularly in LMIC settings.
- Evaluate systemic factors that contribute to inequities in maternal healthcare, and how these disparities can impact maternal health outcomes.

5.1 Introduction

Research interest in intensive care unit (ICU) admission and outcomes has increased. Some determinants as race or socioeconomical status are more often discussed than sex or gender on critical illness, as women have been traditionally excluded from clinical trials [1]. Ensuring equity in healthcare, including perioperative care, is vital. This means providing fair and equal treatment for all individuals, including vulnerable or minority groups, such as pregnant patients.

Despite contemporary policies aimed at promoting health equity, significant disparities in maternal healthcare persist [2]. Fortunately, most women remain healthy during pregnancy and childbirth. Nonetheless, prenatal health is recognized as a crucial component of overall maternal health during pregnancy [3, 4]. Evidence indicates that poor health outcomes during this period are often due to inequitable access to, and limited engagement with, prenatal care services [3, 4]. Inadequate prenatal care has been shown to increase the risk of complications for both the mother and the child, both during pregnancy and in the postpartum period.

The number of women experiencing health complications around childbirth is rising, driven by factors such as advanced maternal age, obesity, and increased comorbidities [5]. Conditions like infection, haemorrhage, and preeclampsia account for more than 60% of critical care admissions in obstetric patients [6]. Some women can deteriorate rapidly, with little or no warning, and may require urgent transfer to a higher level of care [6].

Women who experience acute illness during pregnancy, labour, or the postpartum period must have immediate access to critical care, at the same standard as any other critically ill patient [5]. This care should be delivered by specialized teams with expertise in managing the acutely deteriorating obstetric patient [5]. However, the availability of skilled healthcare professionals and critical care staff may be limited in some settings. Additionally, even intensivists may lack experience in managing obstetric patients [6].

While the critical care environment may not always be the ideal setting for treating obstetric patients around the time of delivery, some patients may receive optimal care in maternity units with trained, experienced personnel [5, 6]. If transfer to an ICU is necessary, it is essential that obstetric care remains available [5].

In summary, the perioperative management and care of critically ill pregnant patients require a multidisciplinary approach. This approach must account for the unique physiological changes of pregnancy, the critical condition of the patient, and the specific competences of the healthcare team.

In this chapter, we analyse challenges in care and the access to critical care, with specific focus on pregnant women and suggest the solutions which can be proposed for the future.

5.2 General Epidemiology and Women Access to the ICU

Several epidemiological studies have highlighted sex-related disparities in ICU admissions and resource utilization. Despite similar severity levels, women often experience lower admission rates compared to men [7–12]. Additionally, certain medical interventions, such as tracheostomy or dialysis, are more frequently administered to men, who also tend to have longer durations of mechanical ventilation [8] and undergo more invasive procedures and treatments [9]. Even sociodemographic factors, such as marital status, have also been identified as influencing differences in care [13], although the underlying reasons are multifactorial and warrant further investigation.

In terms of resource consumption, men have been observed to have higher hospital mortality rates, particularly among postoperative ICU patients. This may be linked to sex-based differences in immune response, potentially modulated by sex hormones [14]. Male gender has been associated with an increased risk of mortality, particularly in the oldest age group (75 years or older) and among patients with relatively low APACHE II scores (<16). Notably, approximately two-thirds of ICU resources were consumed by male patients [14].

Sex hormones may also influence the innate immune response in women, playing a crucial role in ICU admission and outcomes, especially in conditions like shock, trauma, and sepsis. Some studies suggest that women under 50 years of age may have better outcomes in these scenarios, potentially due to the protective effects of oestrogen [15]. However, these differences are complex, as hormonal fluctuations during the menstrual cycle and variations in hormone therapy can influence immune function. These factors remain underexplored.

> **Reflection Point** Given the observed disparities in ICU admissions and resource utilization, it is important to critically examine whether healthcare resources are being allocated in a way that aligns with the principles of equity. Are resources being distributed based on horizontal equity, ensuring equal treatment for equal need, or is there a greater focus on vertical equity, where more intensive care is directed towards those with higher levels of need? This question challenges us to consider how sex-based differences, along with other factors, might influence the fairness and efficiency of healthcare delivery.

5.3 Respiratory Pathology, Gender, and Pregnant Population: What Is Different?

Gender differences in the development and outcomes of acute respiratory distress syndrome (ARDS) have been well-documented. Several factors, including clinical, environmental, genetic, and gender-related differences, may influence the onset of ARDS. Research suggests that women may be more predisposed to developing ARDS following trauma, even after adjusting for age, mechanism of injury, and transfusion rate [16]. In contrast, male patients with ARDS related to COVID-19 have shown higher mortality rates, which may be linked to increased IL-6 production in males and the oestrogen-mediated downregulation of angiotensin-converting enzyme 2 (ACE2) receptors [17].

However, clinical trials investigating supportive treatments in ARDS have predominantly included male participants [18, 19]. In the largest global clinical trial, the LUNG-SAFE trial, a prospective multicentre study involving 50 countries, women were less likely to receive ventilation with low tidal volumes. This difference is likely attributable to women's generally smaller body size, which can complicate the accurate estimation of ideal body weight for ventilation [20]. There is currently no evidence to suggest that susceptibility to ventilator-induced lung injury is more pronounced in either gender [21].

Pregnancy-related complications can lead to development of ARDS and should be considered in the differential diagnosis (pulmonary oedema versus ARDS). These complications include amniotic fluid embolism, tocolytic-induced pulmonary oedema, preeclampsia/eclampsia, and maternal sepsis.

The physiological changes associated with pregnancy play a significant role in the development of ARDS and other related complications. These changes include respiratory alkalosis, decreased chest compliance, diaphragmatic compression from the gravid uterus, and hormonal influences, which collectively reduce functional residual capacity. These factors make ventilating pregnant patients particularly challenging. Additionally, permissive hypercapnia poses an added difficulty, as it must be carefully balanced with the need to maintain adequate uterine and placental perfusion when the baby is still in uterus. Determining the optimal timing for delivery in ARDS patients is also a complex decision [22].

Recommendations for managing ARDS in pregnant patients have largely been extrapolated from non-pregnant populations due to the lack of high-quality data specifically involving pregnant women. The recommended SpO_2 target for pregnant patients is 94%, with an emphasis on providing adequate fetal support while avoiding permissive hypercapnia, as both hypoxia and acidosis can be harmful to the fetus [23].

5.4 Sepsis and Pregnant Patients

Maternal sepsis is a leading cause of ICU admission and accounts for approximately 23% of maternal deaths. In the United States, a study including nearly six million deliveries in the analysis found that maternal sepsis complicates 0.04% of pregnancies [24]. Recognized risk factors for sepsis during pregnancy include white ethnicity, obesity, diabetes mellitus, prolonged active labour, and extended rupture of membranes.

Pregnancy-related immunological changes, such as the downregulation of T-cell lymphocytes, may increase susceptibility to infections like group A Streptococcus, Listeria monocytogenes, and more severe fungal infections [25].

The physiological changes associated with pregnancy can sometimes mask the symptoms of sepsis, potentially leading to delays in the initiation of antibiotic therapy [25].

5.5 Critically Ill Obstetric Patients: Outcome and Research

In the United States, between 200 and 700 women per 100,000 deliveries require ICU admission annually [26]. There are significant disparities in maternal mortality ratios (MMR) based on country income levels. In low- and middle-income countries (LMICs), MMR can reach up to 462 per 100,000, while in high-income countries (HIC), it is as low as 11 per 100,000. However, MMR has been rising in the United States, despite being classified as a high-income country, largely due to factors such as advanced maternal age, obesity, and comorbidities. As a result, ICU admissions in the Unted States and other HICs are expected to increase [27–29].

Inequities in access to care are major contributors to the rising maternal mortality rates in both the United States and the UK [2, 5]. Vulnerable populations, such as Black women, immigrants, and those from socioeconomically deprived areas, are particularly at risk due to limited access to high-quality healthcare. Alarmingly, up to 50% of maternal deaths are considered preventable, with many attributed to postpartum haemorrhage (PPH), hypertension, thromboembolism, and sepsis [30–32].

In recent years, significant research has focused on the ***Modified Early Obstetric Warning Score (MEOWS)***, a scale specifically designed for the pregnant population to facilitate the early detection of maternal deterioration. This tool has been widely used in the UK and internationally and is recommended in the European minimum standards for obstetric anaesthesia and analgesia [33]. Validation studies have shown that MEOWS has a sensitivity of 89%, specificity of 79%, a positive predictive value of 39%, and a negative predictive value of 98% [34]. It is a simple, validated, and effective tool for assessing the severity of the four most common causes of ICU admission in pregnant women: sepsis, cardiac deterioration, hypertension, and postpartum haemorrhage (PPH). The use of MEOWS enables early identification of deteriorating patients and has been associated with improved outcomes [35]. It also allows healthcare providers to anticipate and respond promptly, particularly in cases such as PPH progression [36, 37].

Modified Early Obstetric Warning System (MEOWS) [38] is a physiological scoring system based on **National Early Warning Score (NEWS)**. This tool mainly applies to perinatal areas for early identifying patients who are at risk of deterioration during antepartum, labour and delivery, or postpartum phase. **MEOWS** alert triggers when the required documentation has met the specific criteria.

MEOWS is based on the following assessment parameters and observations:

- Level of Consciousness (AVPU—Alert, Verbal, Pain, & Unresponsive)
- Respiratory Rate
- Oxygen Saturation (SpO2)
- Oxygen Flow Rate
- Heart Rate
- Systolic and Diastolic Blood Pressure (SBP/DBP)
- Temperature
- Urine Output

General Status (Looks Well or Looks unwell)

There is limited evidence regarding the direct impact of ICU admission on maternal outcomes, even though these units provide critically ill obstetric patients with comprehensive, multidisciplinary care, which is focused on both obstetric and familial outcomes. Moreover, research involving critically ill pregnant patients remains scarce, as pregnant women are often excluded from clinical trials.

5.6 Obstetric Anesthesia and Critical Care in LMICs

The issue of maternal mortality in low- and middle-income countries (LMICs) has been extensively discussed by numerous authors [39]. Caesarean delivery and the care of critically ill obstetric patients are crucial services. However, these services are sometimes unavailable or unsafe in LMICs [40, 41].

One of the major challenges in addressing maternal mortality in these regions is combating the "three delays":

- ***First delay: The delay in deciding to seek healthcare***. This is often caused by factors such as lack of knowledge, gender inequities, negative past experiences with the healthcare system, and financial barriers to accessing care.
- ***Second delay: The delay in reaching a healthcare facility***. A significant portion of the population in LMICs lives far from healthcare centres, and transportation logistics can be particularly challenging, especially for critically ill patients requiring urgent care.

- ***Third delay: The delay in receiving appropriate care once the patient arrives at a healthcare facility***. This can be due to infrastructural limitations, inadequate staffing, shortages of essential supplies such as disposables or blood, or the need to transfer the patient to a higher-level facility due to the severity of the medical condition [42]. Such delays can significantly hinder the timely treatment of life-threatening conditions.

The impact of these delays is difficult to quantify, as health information systems in many LMICs are often underdeveloped or non-existent [43].

Reflection Point Severe obstetric emergencies, where rapid response is crucial, are unfortunately common in low- and middle-income countries (LMICs). Most maternal deaths occur during the intrapartum or early postpartum periods, emphasizing the critical need for effective and timely care during these high-risk stages. *How can healthcare systems in LMICs be strengthened to ensure timely, high-quality care for pregnant women, especially during critical moments like childbirth and the postpartum period?*

Staff training and education are critical in reducing or preventing the third delay (the delay in receiving appropriate care once at a healthcare facility) [43].

The early involvement of anaesthesia providers as part of the obstetric team can also help minimize the third delay. Anaesthesia providers should be integrated into decision-making processes related to specific interventions, transfers, and referrals to higher-level care facilities. This inclusion improves team communication and enhances the overall effectiveness of maternal care [43]. However, the quality of anaesthesia varies widely, even within different regions of the same country. Basic infrastructure, such as electricity, water, and medical gases, is often scarce or unreliable. In addition, anaesthesia machines, monitors, and essential medical supplies may be absent, broken, or in short supply, further complicating care delivery [43].

A significant challenge in LMICs is the lack of adequately trained nursing staff, if they are available at all. In some cases, the only anaesthesia provider may be a nurse or even a non-healthcare technician. In certain facilities, there may be no anaesthesia provider present at all [43]. Given these circumstances, the use of neuraxial anaesthesia may not be the optimal decision particularly when a caesarean delivery is required. Arterial hypotension and other complications associated with spinal anaesthesia may be more severe and dangerous in these settings, especially without access to necessary vasopressors or monitoring equipment [42].

Postpartum haemorrhage (PPH) remains the leading cause of maternal mortality in LMICs, with blood resources often being either absent or severely limited. Effective communication between the surgical and anaesthesia teams is crucial. When blood is unavailable, basic interventions, such as maintaining normothermia and using crystalloids and vasopressors, may be lifesaving. In some cases, epinephrine may be the only available vasopressor. Misoprostol is a valuable option for treating uterine atony, as it does not require refrigeration for storage [44].

Although access to pain management is considered a human right in many countries, it remains unaffordable in LMICs due to limited technical and human resources [45].

When resources permit, spinal analgesia during the second stage of labour may be an option. It can also assist during operative deliveries, such as forceps or other instrumental deliveries, reducing pain associated with these procedures. Complications are rare, particularly when low doses are used, making it a relatively safe technique. However, proper training of nursing staff is essential to ensure adequate monitoring of both the mother and the child during the procedure.

The COVID-19 pandemic has added additional challenges to the obstetric patient population. Despite any other concerns, it seems that spinal anaesthesia proved to be a good choice of anaesthesia if feasible, even for Caesarean section for COVID-19 patients, as the results have shown no differences neither in maternal nor in neonatal outcomes [46, 47]. Healthcare system responses to pandemic challenges opened new perspectives and questions of equitable and fair healthcare not only for vulnerable patient populations but global access to treatments that are considered standard of care.

Summary of Recommendations for Critically Ill Pregnant Patients

The principles of perioperative management of critically ill pregnant patients are:

1. Multidisciplinary team approach.
   (a) Involvement of obstetricians, anaesthesiologists, and other needed specialists is crucial to get better outcomes and communication.
   (b) Close communication between the teams: surgical-obstetric team and anaesthesia-critical care team.
2. Physiological changes in pregnancy.
   (a) Keep in mind and be aware of cardiovascular changes, respiratory physiology changes, and haematological-coagulation adaptations or changes related to pregnancy.
3. Anaesthetic considerations.
   (a) A good and careful selection of anaesthetic technique may be vital for sick pregnant women or patients with co-morbidities. A good perioperative evaluation and management are important issues.
   (b) Regional anaesthesia is the gold standard, in most of situations, considering risks and benefits and individualizing the anaesthetic approach as much as possible.
4. Fetal monitoring.
   (a) When appropriate, continuous fetal monitoring is needed during the ICU stay, or periodic monitoring, depending on the mother situation.

   (b) Coordination with neonatologists is needed, especially when it can be expected a preterm delivery.
5. Hemodynamic stability.
   (a) Maternal hemodynamic stability with vasopressors or any other measure is vital to ensure oxygen delivery to the fetus, as utero-placental flow does not have autoregulation and depends on maternal hemodynamics.
   (b) Invasive monitoring may be used when needed, as in any other patient.
6. Postoperative care.
   (a) Pain treatment is essential after surgery, and close monitoring looking for postoperative complications, even more in high-risk patients (obese, hypertense, ageing patients, etc.)
   (b) Monitoring for signs of preterm labour or other complications from the obstetric point of view.

By integrating principles of recommended measures into perioperative and peripartum care and promoting equity, healthcare systems can strive to provide optimal care for all patients, including critically ill pregnant individuals, while ensuring fairness and equality in the delivery of healthcare services.

Proposed Actions

- Enhance education and training for all healthcare professionals involved in the perioperative and critical care of pregnant women, particularly those experiencing acute deterioration. Targeted groups include obstetricians, midwives, obstetric anaesthetists, physicians, intensivists, and critical care nurses. This can be achieved using existing teaching and training resources, as well as updating curricula.
- Foster collaboration between maternity and critical care teams to ensure the optimization of care for critically ill pregnant women, regardless of the care setting. Interdisciplinary communication and teamwork should be prioritized to improve patient outcomes.
- Promote the widespread adoption of early warning systems and any other tools to facilitate the early identification and **timely transfer of pregnant patients to appropriate levels of care.** This approach can help improve maternal outcomes and reduce delays in critical care access.

References

1. Lat TI, McGraw MK, White HD. Gender differences in critical illness and critical care research. Clin Chest Med. 2021;42(3):543–55. https://doi.org/10.1016/j.ccm.2021.04.012. PMID: 34353458; PMCID: PMC8328243
2. Ladak Z, Grewal N, Kim MO, et al. Equity in prenatal healthcare services globally: an umbrella review. BMC Pregnancy Childbirth. 2024;24(1):191. Published 2024 Mar 11. https://doi.org/10.1186/s12884-024-06388-0.
3. WHO. Health topics: maternal health. 2021. Available from: https://www.who.int/health-topics/maternal-health#tab=tab_1. [cited 2021 Dec 15].
4. Buultjens M, Farouque A, Karimi L, Whitby L, Milgrom J, Erbas B. The contribution of group prenatal care to maternal psychological health outcomes: a systematic review. Women Birth. 2021;34:e631–42.
5. https://www.rcoa.ac.uk/sites/default/files/documents/2020-06/EMC-Guidelines2018.pdf
6. Banerjee A, Cantellow S. Maternal critical care: part I. BJA Educ. 2021;21(4):140–7. https://doi.org/10.1016/j.bjae.2020.12.003.
7. Raine R, Goldfrad C, Rowan K, Black N. Influence of patient gender on admission to intensive care. J Epidemiol Community Health. 2002;56(6):418–23. https://doi.org/10.1136/jech.56.6.418. PMID: 12011195; PMCID: PMC1732172
8. Blecha S, Zeman F, Specht S, Lydia Pfefferle A, Placek S, Karagiannidis C, Bein T. Invasiveness of treatment is gender dependent in intensive care: results from a retrospective analysis of 26,711 cases. Anesth Analg. 2021;132(6):1677–83. https://doi.org/10.1213/ANE.0000000000005082.
9. Valentin A, Jordan B, Lang T, Hiesmayr M, Metnitz PG. Gender-related differences in intensive care: a multiple-center cohort study of therapeutic interventions and outcome in critically ill patients. Crit Care Med. 2003;31(7):1901–7. https://doi.org/10.1097/01.CCM.0000069347.78151.50.
10. Fowler RA, Sabur N, Li P, Juurlink DN, Pinto R, Hladunewich MA, Adhikari NK, Sibbald WJ, Martin CM. Sex-and age-based differences in the delivery and outcomes of critical care. CMAJ. 2007;177(12):1513–9. https://doi.org/10.1503/cmaj.071112. Epub 2007 Nov 14. PMID: 18003954; PMCID: PMC2096494
11. Dodek P, Kozak JF, Norena M, Wong H. More men than women are admitted to 9 intensive care units in British Columbia. J Crit Care. 2009;24(4):630.e1–8. https://doi.org/10.1016/j.jcrc.2009.02.010. Epub 2009 May 7
12. Romo H, Amaral AC, Vincent JL. Effect of patient sex on intensive care unit survival. Arch Intern Med. 2004;164(1):61–5. https://doi.org/10.1001/archinte.164.1.61.
13. Sharma RK, Prigerson HG, Penedo FJ, Maciejewski PK. Male-female patient differences in the association between end-of-life discussions and receipt of intensive care near death. Cancer. 2015;121(16):2814–20. https://doi.org/10.1002/cncr.29417. Epub 2015 May 14. PMID: 25975179; PMCID: PMC4529758
14. Reinikainen M, Niskanen M, Uusaro A, Ruokonen E. Impact of gender on treatment and outcome of ICU patients. Acta Anaesthesiol Scand. 2005;49(7):984–90. https://doi.org/10.1111/j.1399-6576.2005.00759.x.
15. Wohltmann CD, Franklin GA, Boaz PW, Luchette FA, Kearney PA, Richardson JD, Spain DA. A multicenter evaluation of whether gender dimorphism affects survival after trauma. Am J Surg. 2001;181(4):297–300. https://doi.org/10.1016/s0002-9610(01)00582-7.
16. Heffernan DS, Dossett LA, Lightfoot MA, Fremont RD, Ware LB, Sawyer RG, May AK. Gender and acute respiratory distress syndrome in critically injured adults: a prospective study. J Trauma. 2011;71(4):878–83. discussion 883-5. doi: https://doi.org/10.1097/TA.0b013e31822c0d31. PMID: 21986736; PMCID: PMC3201740
17. Scully EP, Haverfield J, Ursin RL, Tannenbaum C, Klein SL. Considering how biological sex impacts immune responses and COVID-19 outcomes. Nat Rev Immunol. 2020;20(7):442–7.

https://doi.org/10.1038/s41577-020-0348-8. Epub 2020 June 11. PMID: 32528136; PMCID: PMC7288618
18. Acute Respiratory Distress Syndrome Network, Brower RG, Matthay MA, Morris A, Schoenfeld D, Thompson BT, Wheeler A. Ventilation with lower tidal volumes as compared with traditional tidal volumes for acute lung injury and the acute respiratory distress syndrome. N Engl J Med. 2000;342(18):1301–8. https://doi.org/10.1056/NEJM200005043421801.
19. Guérin C, Reignier J, Richard JC, Beuret P, Gacouin A, Boulain T, Mercier E, Badet M, Mercat A, Baudin O, Clavel M, Chatellier D, Jaber S, Rosselli S, Mancebo J, Sirodot M, Hilbert G, Bengler C, Richecoeur J, Gainnier M, Bayle F, Bourdin G, Leray V, Girard R, Baboi L, Ayzac L, PROSEVA Study Group. Prone positioning in severe acute respiratory distress syndrome. N Engl J Med. 2013;368(23):2159–68. https://doi.org/10.1056/NEJMoa1214103. Epub 2013 May 20
20. L'her E, Martin-Babau J, Lellouche F. Accuracy of height estimation and tidal volume setting using anthropometric formulas in an ICU Caucasian population. Ann Intensive Care. 2016;6(1):55. https://doi.org/10.1186/s13613-016-0154-4. Epub 2016 June 21. PMID: 27325410; PMCID: PMC4916127
21. López-Alonso I, Amado-Rodriguez L, López-Martínez C, Huidobro C, Albaiceta GM. Sex susceptibility to ventilator-induced lung injury. Intensive Care Med Exp. 2019;7(1):7. https://doi.org/10.1186/s40635-019-0222-9. PMID: 30635805; PMCID: PMC6329690
22. Schnettler WT, Al Ahwel Y, Suhag A. Severe acute respiratory distress syndrome in coronavirus disease 2019-infected pregnancy: obstetric and intensive care considerations. Am J Obstet Gynecol MFM. 2020;2(3):100120. https://doi.org/10.1016/j.ajogmf.2020.100120. Epub 2020 Apr 14. PMID: 32363337; PMCID: PMC7194528
23. Cole DE, Taylor TL, McCullough DM, Shoff CT, Derdak S. Acute respiratory distress syndrome in pregnancy. Crit Care Med. 2005;33(10 Suppl):S269–78. https://doi.org/10.1097/01.ccm.0000182478.14181.da.
24. Hensley MK, Bauer ME, Admon LK, Prescott HC. Incidence of maternal sepsis and sepsis-related maternal deaths in the United States. JAMA. 2019;322(9):890–2. https://doi.org/10.1001/jama.2019.9818. PMID: 31479129; PMCID: PMC6724160
25. Pietropaoli AP, Glance LG, Oakes D, Fisher SG. Gender differences in mortality in patients with severe sepsis or septic shock. Gend Med. 2010;7(5):422–37. https://doi.org/10.1016/j.genm.2010.09.005. PMID: 21056869; PMCID: PMC3322379
26. Guntupalli KK, Hall N, Karnad DR, Bandi V, Belfort M. Critical illness in pregnancy: part I: an approach to a pregnant patient in the ICU and common obstetric disorders. Chest. 2015;148(4):1093–104. https://doi.org/10.1378/chest.14-1998.
27. Alkema L, Chou D, Hogan D, Zhang S, Moller AB, Gemmill A, Fat DM, Boerma T, Temmerman M, Mathers C, Say L. United Nations maternal mortality estimation inter-agency group collaborators and technical advisory group. Global, regional, and national levels and trends in maternal mortality between 1990 and 2015, with scenario-based projections to 2030: a systematic analysis by the UN maternal mortality estimation inter-agency group. Lancet. 2016;387(10017):462–74. https://doi.org/10.1016/S0140-6736(15)00838-7. Epub 2015 Nov 13. PMID: 26584737; PMCID: PMC5515236
28. https://www.who.int/news-room/fact-sheets/detail/maternal-mortality. Accesed Nov 2023.
29. https://www.cdc.gov/reproductivehealth/maternal-mortality/erase-mm/data-mmrc.html. Accesed Nov 2023.
30. Farquhar C, Sadler L, Masson V, Bohm G, Haslam A. Beyond the numbers: classifying contributory factors and potentially avoidable maternal deaths in New Zealand, 2006–2009. Am J Obstet Gynecol. 2011;205(4):331.e1–8. https://doi.org/10.1016/j.ajog.2011.07.044. Epub 2011 July 30
31. Saucedo M, Deneux-Tharaux C, Bouvier-Colle MH. French National Experts Committee on maternal mortality. Ten years of confidential inquiries into maternal deaths in France, 1998–2007. Obstet Gynecol. 2013;122(4):752–60. https://doi.org/10.1097/AOG.0b013e31829fc38c.

32. Creanga AA, Berg CJ, Syverson C, Seed K, Bruce FC, Callaghan WM. Pregnancy-related mortality in the United States, 2006-2010. Obstet Gynecol. 2015;125(1):5–12. https://doi.org/10.1097/AOG.0000000000000564.
33. Guasch E, Brogly N, Mercier FJ, Ioscovich A, Weiniger CF, Lucas N, Chassard D, Kranke P, Whitaker D, Geldner G, Sabelnikovs O, de Robertis E. European minimum standards for obstetric analgesia and anaesthesia departments: an experts' consensus. Eur J Anaesthesiol. 2020;37(12):1115–25. https://doi.org/10.1097/EJA.0000000000001362.
34. Singh S, McGlennan A, England A, Simons R. A validation study of the CEMACH recommended modified early obstetric warning system (MEOWS). Anaesthesia. 2012;67(1):12–8. https://doi.org/10.1111/j.1365-2044.2011.06896.x. Epub 2011 Nov 9. Erratum in: Anaesthesia. 2012 Apr;67(4):453
35. Zuckerwise LC, Lipkind HS. Maternal early warning systems-towards reducing preventable maternal mortality and severe maternal morbidity through improved clinical surveillance and responsiveness. Semin Perinatol. 2017;41(3):161–5. https://doi.org/10.1053/j.semperi.2017.03.005. Epub 2017 Apr 14
36. Baek MS, Son J, Huh JW, Lim CM, Koh Y, Won HS, Shim JY, Hong SB. Medical emergency team may reduce obstetric intensive care unit admissions. J Obstet Gynaecol Res. 2017;43(1):106–13. https://doi.org/10.1111/jog.13177. Epub 2016 Oct 20
37. Skupski DW, Brady D, Lowenwirt IP, Sample J, Lin SN, Lohana R, Eglinton GS. Improvement in outcomes of major obstetric hemorrhage through systematic change. Obstet Gynecol. 2017;130(4):770–7. https://doi.org/10.1097/AOG.0000000000002207.
38. https://cstcernerhelp.healthcarebc.ca/Workflows/MEOWS/Modified_Early_Obstetric_Warning_System_(MEOWS).htm
39. Guasch E, Brogly N, Gilsanz F. Teaching and learning obstetric anaesthesia in low- and middle-income countries: current situation and perspectives. Curr Anesthesiol Rep. 2023;13(2):76–82. https://doi.org/10.1007/s40140-023-00557-1. Epub 2023 Apr 19. PMID: 37168832; PMCID: PMC10113969
40. Ronsmans C, Graham WJ. Lancet maternal survival series steering group. Maternal mortality: who, when, where, and why. Lancet. 2006;368(9542):1189–200. https://doi.org/10.1016/S0140-6736(06)69380-X.
41. Meara JG, Leather AJ, Hagander L, Alkire BC, Alonso N, Ameh EA, Bickler SW, Conteh L, Dare AJ, Davies J, Mérisier ED, El-Halabi S, Farmer PE, Gawande A, Gillies R, Greenberg SL, Grimes CE, Gruen RL, Ismail EA, Kamara TB, Lavy C, Lundeg G, Mkandawire NC, Raykar NP, Riesel JN, Rodas E, Rose J, Roy N, Shrime MG, Sullivan R, Verguet S, Watters D, Weiser TG, Wilson IH, Yamey G, Yip W. Global surgery 2030: evidence and solutions for achieving health, welfare, and economic development. Lancet. 2015;386(9993):569–624. https://doi.org/10.1016/S0140-6736(15)60160-X. Epub 2015 Apr 26
42. Cavallaro FL, Marchant TJ. Responsiveness of emergency obstetric care systems in low- and middle-income countries: a critical review of the "third delay". Acta Obstet Gynecol Scand. 2013;92(5):496–507. https://doi.org/10.1111/aogs.12071. Epub 2013 Feb 12
43. Bishop D, van Dyk D, Dyer RA. Safe obstetric anaesthesia in low- and middle-income countries-a perspective from Africa. BJA Educ. 2023;23(11):432–9. https://doi.org/10.1016/j.bjae.2023.07.003. Epub 2023 Sept 9. PMID: 37876763; PMCID: PMC10591126
44. Weeks A, Faúndes A. Misoprostol in obstetrics and gynecology. Int J Gynaecol Obstet. 2007;99(Suppl 2):S156–9. https://doi.org/10.1016/j.ijgo.2007.09.003. Epub 2007 Oct 25
45. Schnittger T. Regional anaesthesia in developing countries. Anaesthesia. 2007;62(Suppl 1):44–7. https://doi.org/10.1111/j.1365-2044.2007.05297.x.
46. Ababneh O, Alrabayah M, El-Share' AI, Bsisu I, Bahar Y, Dabousi B, Sandoqa A, AlWreikat D, Qatawneh A. Perioperative outcomes in COVID-19 obstetric patients undergoing spinal anesthesia for cesarean section: a prospective observational study. Healthcare (Basel). 2021;10(1):23. https://doi.org/10.3390/healthcare10010023. PMID: 35052187; PMCID: PMC8774980
47. Ioscovich A, Guasch E, Brogly N, Shatalin D, Manrique-Muñoz S, Sánchez Royo ME, Zimro S, Ginosar Y, Lages N, Weinstein J, Berkenstadt H, Greenberger C, Lazutkin A, Izakson A,

Ioscovich D, Orbach-Zinger S, Weiniger CF. Peripartum anesthetic management of women with SARS-CoV-2 infection in eight medical centers across three European countries: prospective cohort observation study. J Matern Fetal Neonatal Med. 2022;35(25):7756–63. https://doi.org/10.1080/14767058.2021.1937105. Epub 2021 June 9

Non-pregnancy-Related Emergencies in Critically Ill and Surgical Female Patients

6

Pascale Gruber, Bethany Gwyther, and Alexandra M. Hogan

Key Points from the Editors

- Gender differences in life experiences, behaviours, and life events influence how individuals interact with the healthcare system, which can impact their access to care and ultimately affect outcomes.
- Disparities in outcomes for women in critical care and surgical settings persist. These differences may stem from **pathophysiological variations between sexes**, which are often overlooked in clinical decision-making, as well as **systemic biases** within healthcare practices and policies.
- There is a significant gap in research concerning the optimal care for women in critical care and surgery. This gap is largely due to the historical underrepresentation of sex and gender differences in clinical studies. Biological factors influencing care and outcomes need to be better explored in the future (Gender medicine).

P. Gruber (✉)
The Royal Marsden NHS Foundation Trust, London, UK

B. Gwyther
Whittington Health NHS Trust, London, UK
e-mail: bethany.gwyther2@nhs.net

A. M. Hogan
Salisbury Hospital Foundation Trust, Salisbury, UK

School of Health Sciences, University of Southampton, Salisbury, UK
e-mail: Alexandra.Hogan2@nhs.net

V. Neskovic, F. Rubulotta (eds.), *Diversity, Gender Equity and Inclusion in Critical Care and Perioperative Medicine*,
https://doi.org/10.1007/978-3-031-86286-1_6

Main Objectives

After reading this chapter, you will be able to:

- Discuss non-pregnancy-related emergencies in women who are critically ill or post-surgery and describe differences in epidemiology, presentation, management, and both short- and long-term outcomes.
- Distinguish the pathophysiological variations and disease prognosis in women, and list factors that affect outcomes in non-pregnancy-related emergencies.
- Identify areas for improvement in patient management within critical care and surgery, with a focus on improving outcome for women patients.

6.1 Introduction

The impact of pregnancy on women's health is undoubtedly significant and has been covered in a previous chapter. However, there are a vast number of non-pregnancy-related emergencies impacting women, with nearly 60,000 female patients admitted to the intensive care unit (ICU) in the United Kingdom in 2021 alone, with around a third of these coming directly from operating theatres [1].

Globally, there are important differences in lifelong health trajectories between men and women; the average life expectancy gap between men and women currently lies at 4.6 years, with women outliving men, yet spending longer living with disability [2]. Against this background, superimposed acute health issues vary in presentation and severity between men and women.

Within this chapter, we will discuss examples of non-pregnancy-related emergencies in women, in both critically ill and post-surgical patients. While many of these clinical scenarios are not unique to women, there are meaningful differences in the epidemiology, presentation, management, and short- and long-term outcomes. In addition, cross-cutting key themes will be addressed, and these include (1) the relationship between women and their healthcare providers, including their psychological adaptation to becoming a patient; (2) the representation of women in relevant research and, fundamental to this, their inclusion in the development and validation of commonly used assessment tools; and finally, (3) the pathophysiological variation and disease prognosis in women.

6.2 Gender Differences in Critical Care Admission and Outcomes

ICU admission is determined by clinical need; however, gender can influence ICU utilisation. One gender may typically present with more severe disease or have a higher risk-adjusted mortality, warranting ICU admission. However, other factors such as socio-cultural differences or clinician's gender bias may play an important role [3]. Much of the literature reports a male predominance in ICU admissions however the data is incongruous [4, 5].

Similarly, published data in the ICU literature is heterogenous with regard to mortality across genders; individual studies have often demonstrated a small excess mortality amongst women admitted to ICU [5–7], yet few studies have made a definitive conclusion. A recent meta-analysis by Modra et al. did find that, while women accounted for a lower proportion of admissions than men, risk-adjusted mortality was higher amongst them (OR 1.25 95% CI 1.03–1.50) [8].

Several studies have explored differences in the treatment of women, throughout their journey as patient in critical care. Studies in both Austria and Canada have shown that women were less likely to be admitted to the ICU [4, 5]. Once admitted, evidence suggests that men may receive more aggressive treatment than women; a 2021 meta-analysis demonstrated women were less likely than men to receive invasive mechanical ventilation and renal replacement therapy after adjustment for illness severity and other confounders [8]. Similarly, Blecha et al demonstrated that male patients were more likely to undergo tracheostomy, dialysis, extracorporeal membrane oxygenation and pulmonary catheter insertion despite similar severity of illness [9]. Furthermore, it appears that women are more likely to have treatment limitation decisions [10–14]. For example, female sex has been shown to be an independent predictor of treatment limitation decisions in patients with sepsis [15, 16].

While most intensive care patients survive initial admission, many do not recover to the same level of health they had before. There are few studies looking at gender differences in longer term morbidity and mortality after ICU admission. A prospective study investigated 1-year mortality for ICU patients and did not show any significant gender differences in mortality [17]. However, another way of looking at the resultant morbidity of critical care is post-intensive care syndrome (PICS), which describes worsened physical and mental health, and cognitive impairment following a stay in ICU. This appears to impact women disproportionately to men; Lee et al demonstrated that those of female sex are nearly twice as likely to suffer physical impairment following ICU admission, and three times as likely to have resultant worsened mental health. In fact, female sex was associated with a higher risk of negative psychological outcomes than all other risk factors, apart from previous mental health problems [18].

A secondary analysis of the Bringing to Light the Risk Factors and Incidence of Neuropsychological Dysfunction in ICU survivors (BRAIN-ICU) showed an **increase daily living disability, worsening of physical function related quality of life, more depressive symptoms, and higher reported rates of post-traumatic stress disorder** in females at 3 months following ICU discharge. At 12 months, trauma symptoms and reduction of global physical function **remained worse** in women [19].

Disease severity and prognostication scales are commonly used in the ICU setting. For example, the APACHE (Acute Physiology and Chronic Health Evaluation) scoring system considers age and several other important markers of disease severity including chronic health conditions, blood test markers, and common observations including heart rate and blood pressure. Combined, these markers can be used to predict mortality rate for certain groups of patients. The APACHE score does not distinguish between gender but has been included in some critical care studies that have focused on gender differences. For example, Kim and colleagues described a cohort of 103 patients in critical care with stress-induced cardiomyopathy [20]. Whilst the APACHE score did not differ between men and women, there were important differences in disease presentation and recovery; men were more likely to present following an 'acute medical illnesses' whereas women were significantly more likely to present following 'emotional stress'. Interestingly, women were found to more likely present with chest pain, in contrast to the published literature on acute coronary syndromes [21]. All-cause mortality at follow-up was higher in men with a low ejection fraction at 2 months, whereas an initial high APACHE score was significant for women. Thus, despite the APACHE score initially being similar, there were some notable differences between the presentation of men and women with this condition. The authors highlighted that further studies are warranted to understand the gender differences in antecedent stressors leading to this condition. If research focuses on assessment tools without considering whether gender is accounted for, we lose the opportunity to learn from what may be important differences in patient care.

> There is evidence to suggest women may be less likely to receive intensive care treatment, and when they are admitted, may be more likely to die, or have poor long-term outcomes. Furthermore, some research that has guided ICU practice has neglected gender differences, perhaps due to assumptions that it is a variable already accounted for in the validation of commonly used assessment tools and thus not explored further.

6.3 Gender Differences in Surgical Outcomes

It is estimated that the average person undergoes nine surgical procedures over the course of their life. The nature of these procedures will differ between genders, with the most common procedure undertaken by women being caesarean section [22]. A 2022 European Union report also showed an increase in minimally invasive procedures, for example, laparoscopic hysterectomies, in women [23].

When considering surgical outcomes and gender it is imperative to keep in mind the fast, evolving landscape of surgical techniques and the impact of novel interventions. Assessing possible differences in surgical outcomes between sexes is a subject fraught with difficulty. For some procedures, such as cardiac surgery, female sex appears to be an independent risk factor for mortality [24, 25]. This difference is not universal, with male patients appearing to have higher mortality in several other areas [26–28]. However, when we look for more detailed surgical outcome data, including differences in morbidity, we often find a lack of information; in part because women are simply not as frequently included in surgical trials [29, 30]. Take carotid procedures as an example; while women experience worse disability and higher mortality following an ischaemic stroke, they are underrepresented in trials of carotid revascularisation [31]. This not only impacts clinical practice, but also the way in which we are able to discuss high-risk procedures with women and in the ability to obtain informed consent. This is by no means an issue unique to surgery, and rather permeates through medical research and other areas of evidence-based medical practice [32, 33].

Reflection Point How does the way we talk to women about high-risk procedures, especially when explaining risks and getting their consent, show bigger problems in healthcare? How do issues in medical research and practices make these problems worse? What can we do to improve communication and understanding, especially in urgent situations?

The importance of the relationship between women and their healthcare providers is an important area of focus in the context of surgery. A large population-based study of 1,320,108 patients and 2937 surgeons by Wallis et al examined patient-surgeon sex discordance on adverse outcomes including complications, 30-day post-operative mortality and readmission rate. Subgroup analysis of four categories of biological sex-dyads revealed a higher rate of adverse outcomes when female patients were treated by male surgeons [34]. This occurred despite possible mediating factors including surgeon experience and patient age. The authors highlight two possible explanations. Firstly, male physicians' underappreciation of symptoms reported by women, and they cite evidence in support of this from the cardiac and pain literature, and, secondly, women under-reporting their symptoms to male physicians. Either way, this study suggests that addressing social, psychological, and communication barriers to women's access to and acceptance of improved healthcare is essential. This study raises several additional questions. For example, whilst the length of stay for all types of surgeries was shorter for women across all surgery types and this may in part be accounted for by differences in complication rate, it would be of interest to understand why women might leave hospital sooner post-operatively. The possibility of wider socio-cultural influences on their healthcare providers' decision-making could be informative. For example, there is the possibility that women are under a real or perceived sense of pressure to return to everyday life. This study reflects another important consideration, namely that related to the surgeons themselves. The surgical profession remains subject to a deep gender bias, with only 14.7% of surgical consultants in England being female [35].

The study by Wallis and colleagues described above, like many others, relied on standard markers of surgical outcomes to underpin its methodology. For example, 30-day mortality and risk scoring systems. These may be subject and vulnerable to bias. For example, Mayhew et al demonstrated a vulnerability to bias in ratings given to children and to women in the American Society of Anaesthesiology (ASA) classification [36]. Similarly, use of POSSUM and APACHE as a tool in studies may impact on the reporting of outcomes.

We do know that women can have a different experience of surgical intervention compared to men. For example, they are more likely to be anxious pre-operatively [37]. There are also differences in the recognition and management of post-operative pain [38–40]. These differences in patient journey are not trivial and could conceivably be a barrier to the provision of high-quality surgical care. Wallis et al suggested potential avenues for research regarding unrecognised gender bias in surgical outcomes [34].

6.4 Exploring Gender Differences in Outcomes in Critical Care and Post-operative Patients

Care of a female patient on the ICU and post-operatively requires the healthcare professional to have competencies in the management of gender-specific conditions such as maternity care (e.g., eclampsia, amniotic fluid embolism, acute fatty liver, post-partum haemorrhage), and gynaecological conditions (e.g., gynaecological cancers, endometriosis) but also an appreciation of the difference is incidence, presentation, and management of common medical conditions.

However, as explored above, there are discrepancies in outcomes for women admitted to critical care or undergoing surgery. It is next important to consider why these differences exist. In this section, we address the multifactorial and interconnected aspects of this area of health inequality.

6.4.1 Endocrine Differences

There is evidence of a biological difference in physiological response to the surgical insult and critical illness between men and women. Sex has been found to influence the expression, progression, and outcome for many common conditions, including severe infection and sepsis [41, 42]. Preclinical data indicates that oestrogen may play a beneficial role in the pathophysiology and recovery from critical illness and surgery [43–45]. It appears to have an antioxidant and protective effect in trauma, sepsis, and major haemorrhage 46–48). Oestrogen has been shown to preserve cardiovascular and immunological function and tolerance to severe hypoxia [46, 47]. In experimental models of *E. coli* administration, females have demonstrated a greater pro-inflammatory response and norepinephrine sensitivity [43]. Hormonal manipulation in animal models has been shown to reduce sepsis-related mortality in males [48]. Oestrogens reduce chemotaxis and activation of neutrophils and pulmonary injury following massive haemorrhage [49]. Administration of oestrogen receptor agonists has been shown to preserve gastrointestinal mucosal barrier function and improve outcomes in in-vitro models of sepsis [50]. Despite the advantages shown in the preclinical setting, the findings in epidemiological studies have been inconsistent. Some studies have indicated that women of premenopausal age have a higher ICU survival, better physiological response to trauma and outcome following cardiac arrest whilst other studies have failed to demonstrate this advantage [5, 13, 51]. An important confounder in studies where sex is a categorical variable is that hormonal levels may vary considerably during menstrual cycles and menopause and are modifiable with diet and exercise.

Oestrogen and other sex-related hormones may partially explain differences in how individuals respond to critical illness and surgery. However, since critical illness and surgery involve a wide range of complex underlying factors, it is unlikely that biological differences related to sex alone can fully account for these variations or apply uniformly in all cases. Other factors need to be considered.

6.4.2 Respiratory System Differences

There are several differences in respiratory physiology between men and women: From the hormonal impact of testosterone, which appears to reduce the response to histamine in the airway, to the anatomical, with fewer alveoli for the number of airways in boys, resulting in a lower expiratory flow rate. However, the real-world implications of these differences are unclear, in part due to the predominance of research performed in men [52].

Acute respiratory distress syndrome (ARDS) is a common reason for ICU admission. However, gender, as a factor in the development of ARDS has not been well-studied. The recent COVID-19 pandemic demonstrated a male bias in mortality with higher incidence of ARDS and ARDS-related mortality in males. This has been attributed to higher IL-6 and IL-18 production, alongside oestrogen-related down-regulation of angiotensin-converting enzyme 2 receptors [53]. These findings have been mirrored in the past; a higher mortality was also seen in males with ARDS secondary to Severe Acute Respiratory Syndrome (SARS) and Middle East Respiratory Syndrome (MERS-CoV) [54, 55]. In contrast, female trauma patients were found more likely than men to develop ARDS, despite adjusting for age, mechanism of injury, injury severity, and blood product transfusion [56]. Overall, gender bias in the development of ARDS has not been shown consistently in epidemiologic studies, but male sex does seem to confer a higher risk of ARDS-related mortality. In the management of ARDS, analysis of ARDS network trials has showed that women are more likely to receive ventilation with tidal volumes higher than 6 ml/kg [57]. This has been attributed to lower body mass indices seen in women.

6.4.3 Gender Differences in Infection, Inflammation, and Sepsis

Evidence shows that there may be an increase in male predominance for admission to ICU with septic shock [58]. Immunologically, androgens have been shown to have immunosuppressive and oestradiol immunoprotective effects. Data regarding the outcome of sepsis is however conflicting with some studies showing an increase in mortality for female patients, others showing an increase in mortality in male patients and some showing no difference [28, 59–61]. A quarter of maternal deaths are due to sepsis with Group A *Streptococcus* as one of the most common causes of infection [62]. Changes in pregnancy and the down-regulation of T cell activity predispose pregnant patients to a higher risk of infection. Regarding sepsis management, studies have shown that female patients are less likely to receive dialysis and mechanical ventilation during ICU admission for sepsis and septic shock and are more likely to have a delay in the administration of antibiotics [63, 64]. Manipulation of hormonal status in septic patients has been tried in pre-clinical studies however the benefit in sepsis is yet to be determined [48].

The flux of female sex hormones during puberty, pregnancy, and menopause has a substantial impact on both the innate and adaptive immune system. This is associated with the female predominance of autoimmune conditions [65]; 80% of autoimmune diagnoses are in women [66]. In extreme cases, the primary immune disorder may necessitate hospital and ICU admission, or surgical intervention. However, more commonly, long-term immunosuppression can have an impact on the risk of infection, and recovery from ICU or post-operatively.

6.4.4 Cardiovascular System Differences

Cardiovascular anatomy and physiology differ between men and women. Male hearts are larger than female, but differences in important parameters are not fully accounted for by allometric scaling. Female hearts have a larger ejection fraction and larger contractile strains but produce lower cardiac output [67].

Cardiovascular disease and cardiac health influence both surgical outcomes and survival from critical illness. Studies have shown women experience acute coronary syndromes (ACS) differently to men, reflecting in atypical presentations of chest pain. In 2007 a review of 69 studies conducted between 1970 and 2005 described a disproportionate lack of ACS symptoms in women compared to men, but concluded that sex-specific public health messaging was not warranted time [68]. Over a decade later in 2022, authors still note the persistence of gender inequality in the management of ACS generally [69]. The reasons for this are multifactorial and include hormonal changes particularly around the time of menopause, as well as underlying physiological differences in prevalence of metabolic syndrome, and, more specifically, smaller coronary vessel size and greater incidence of small vessel disease [70].

Part of the problem may also be related to bias in the assessment tools employed to determine the severity of cardiac disease. For example, in 2022, it was demonstrated that early iterations of the GRACE score (Global Registry of Acute Coronary

Events 2.0) discriminated in-hospital death following non-ST elevation myocardial infarction significantly better in men than in women ($p<0.0001$; 420,781 patients in total) [71], suggesting that post-ACS complications could have been missed in many women during this time despite the increasing number of studies highlighting gender differences in ACS presentation. However, this was rectified with the development of GRACE 3.0, allowing women with higher risk of complications following ACS to be better recognised.

In summary, cardiovascular disease can be a complicating or a presenting factor in women requiring surgery or critical care. There is evidence that the presentation and management of cardiovascular disease in women can differ from that in men. Less is understood about those differences manifest in the context of emergency surgery and critical care.

6.4.5 Frailty and Fragility

Frailty is defined as an increased state of vulnerability from an ageing-associated decline in reserve and function [72]. As discussed earlier, women experience a prolonged period of "unhealthy" life years when compared to men, due to a widening gap between life expectancy, and healthy life expectancy. This, coupled with numerous interacting biological and sociocultural factors, has led to increased rates of frailty amongst women [38].

There are specific examples of this. For example, 70% of osteoporotic fractures occur in women [73]. Smaller bone and muscle mass contribute to this as well as accelerated bone loss after menopause caused by decreasing oestrogen levels. As such, three-quarters of hip fractures occur in women [74]. The medical complications of hip fracture and subsequent surgery are well known in numerous studies, with a mortality at 1 year estimated at 14-36% [75].

Furthermore, the lifetime frequency of Alzheimer's disease is almost twice as high in women compared to men regardless of age [76]. Dementia is an independent risk factor for poor post-operative outcomes; one 2018 study demonstrated a nearly 50% increased risk of post-operative mortality in patients with dementia compared to matched controls [77].

6.4.6 Pharmacokinetic and Pharmacodynamic Differences

When we look at the medications given; there are pharmaco-kinetic and pharmacodynamic sex differences, with associated variations of therapeutic effects and side effect profiles. Biological sex can affect drug absorption, distribution, metabolism, and elimination. Body fat composition, total blood, plasma and red blood cell volumes, extra cellar water, protein binding, glomerular filtration rate, and membrane receptor sensitivity differ between women and men. Women have a greater body fat composition, lower circulating blood volume, lower plasma volume, and lower volume of distribution [78]. Oestrogen increases the levels of serum-binding globulins

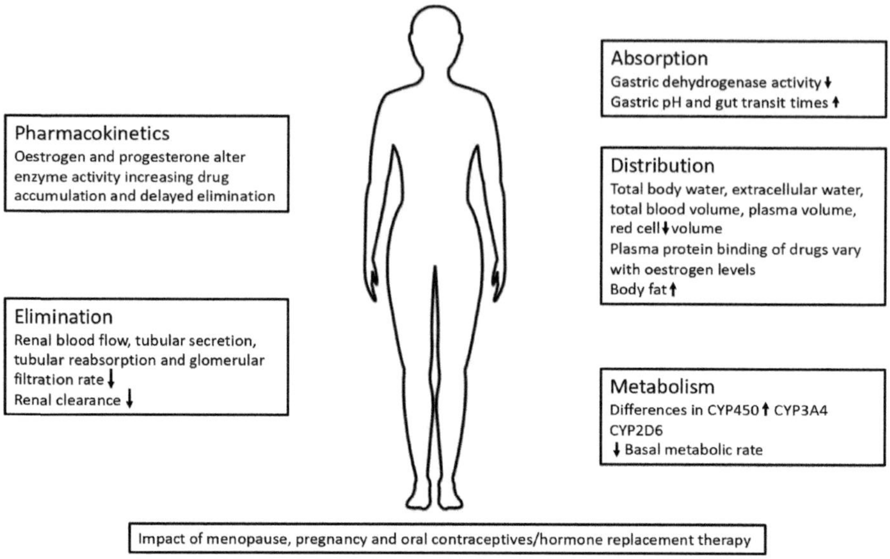

Fig. 6.1 Gender differences in pharmacokinetics and pharmacodynamics

(e.g., sex-hormone-binding globulin, corticosteroid-binding globulin, and thyroxine-binding globulin). Hepatic clearance of drugs is determined by liver blood flow and CYP450 enzymes, with a higher activity in females for CYP3A4 and CYP2D6. Renal blood flow, tubular secretion, and glomerular filtration are all greater in men compared to women even after adjusting for body surface area. Women also have a 1.5 times greater risk of developing adverse drug reactions and are more likely to be on concomitant medications.

The use of enzyme-inducing medications may compromise the efficiency of hormonal contraceptives resulting in an increasing rate of unplanned pregnancies [79]. Menstrual health can be affected by hospital admission with increasing rate of menstrual disturbances reported in women following COVID-19 and other infections thought to be a disruption of the interaction between hypothalamus, pituitary, ovaries, uterus, prostaglandins but also vitamin depletion (Vit C, D, B6) and stressors [80]. However, there is very little data looking at the impact of fertility following hospital admission (Fig. 6.1).

6.4.7 Sociocultural Factors and Gender Biases

Aside from biological sex differences, sociocultural gender differences can impact on the management and outcome of ICU and surgical patients. People of different genders experience life in different ways, exhibit different behaviours, life events and this can lead to different interactions with the healthcare system which may impact on patient outcomes. For example, early claims that excess male COVID-19 deaths were due to biological sex differences with male patients showing higher level of innate immune cytokines such as IL-8, IL-18 and monocytes failed to take account of important social candidate causes such as patterns of occupational exposure, compliance with mask wearing and handwashing, and access to healthcare. Reports in other medical specialities such as cardiovascular medicine have shown non-biological differences contributing to variations in outcomes [81, 82]. Socioeconomic factors may also play a role with women often having less direct access to healthcare due to factors such as insurance, healthcare costs and affordability, illiteracy, social norms, advocacy, and concerns about caregiver (childcare and eldercare) impact.

Other socio-cultural factors need to be considered when caring for the female patient. Women are at higher risk of **domestic violence, sexual abuse** which often present with **anxiety and depression** and clinician should be alert to these signs [83]. Women are often the **primary childcare and eldercare provider**, and this may require the engagement of community services at an early stage. Finally, culturally sensitive issues need to be considered when caring for the female patient with **some cultural limitations for personal care with some religions** [84].

Reflection Point Culturally sensitive issues can affect the communication and relationship between professionals and women patients. Considering migrations and different religious backgrounds, how can we empower professionals to deliver fair and personalised care?

Clinician gender bias may also play a role in patient-clinician communication styles, nonverbal communication, and power dynamics. A systematic review in the general population demonstrated that clinicians do hold implicit biases [85] For example, women are more likely to be undertreated for pain than men [86]. However, studies in the ICU settings have been limited. A survey of over 1000 ICU doctors from 75 countries failed to demonstrate any difference in the approach to ICU triage between female and male patients [12].

An analysis of the Intensive Care National Audit and Research Centre (ICNARC) case mix program by Raine et al showed no evidence of gender differences in case mix on admissions or mortality for patients with cardiac arrhythmias, chronic obstructive airways disease, asthma, self-poisoning, or seizures, however there was horizontal inequity (unequal use for equal need) in female patients with myocardial infarction and with neurological bleeding [3]. Vertical equity, referring to the concept that patients with greater needs should receive more treatment, was not achieved for male patients with pneumonia and ventricular failure and for women with primary brain injury [3]. The reason for the gender disparity in intensity of treatment remains unclear. However, it aligns with findings from other medical specialities such as cardiovascular, oncology and renal medicine. A study by Sharma et al demonstrated that male patients with advanced cancer were more likely to receive aggressive, non-beneficial care in the ICU than women with advanced malignancies [87]. Possible reasons could be the absence of decisional support or advocacy when female patients are critically ill due to higher rates of widowhood, gender bias by clinicians or merely that clinicians could be responding to differences in treatment intensity preferred by women and men, however, none of these theories have been validated [88]. This reflects a complex interplay of physiologic and sociocultural factors.

6.4.8 Pain Management

Pain is a symptom of a wide range of medical conditions, with an estimated 78% of emergency department attendances due to pain [89]. However, pain is a gendered experience; with the severity of pain often underestimated in women due to gender stereotypes and bias of carers and clinicians [90]. Several studies have demonstrated higher rates of post-operative pain amongst women, for a variety of procedure types, with higher post-operative analgesic requirements [40, 91]. While it is hard to quantify pain within the ICU, a large multi-centre study identified that nearly half of intensive care patients had significant pain at 3 months [92]. Hence, pain reflects an important outcome measure for the treatments provided in emergency surgical and critical care interventions. To effectively manage our patient's pain, regardless of gender, it is essential to increase awareness of gender norms in clinical practice and academia [90].

6.4.9 Rehabilitation

Ott et al performed a large scoping review exploring the impact of sex and gender on rehabilitation. This demonstrated that the utilisation of rehabilitation is generally lower amongst women, and those women who did access rehabilitation typically showed less physical and functional improvements than men participants [93]. Several patient factors caused this, including caregiving and familial responsibilities. This reduced access and utilisation of rehabilitation services may contribute to some reduced long-term outcomes discussed earlier in the chapter.

6.5 Conclusions and the Future

In this chapter, we have discussed emergencies in critically ill and surgical female patients. We have addressed differences in epidemiology and outcomes, and have also addressed some of the complex, interacting multi-factorial causes. However, we remain a long way from understanding the biological differences between the male and female sex binary. Furthermore, lack of inclusion means there is also limited research available regarding trans and non-binary individuals.

An understanding on difference in sex-based differences in ICU utilisation and post-ICU and post-surgical outcomes is an important area of future research. An understanding of the biological but also non-biological drivers deserves greater recognition and investigation. A suggested way to launch such an investigation was highlighted by Chen et al who recommended the use of the "5 Whys" technique to identify the system causes of the disparities in care after which factors that can be modified and targeted for improvement [94].

Finally, a greater voice of women's experience in the healthcare system and a universal drive towards improving the quality and accessibility of information and education on women's health is required, ensuring that healthcare systems understand and are responsive to women's needs, support research, and use of evidence-based data. This will enable us to improve and promote women's health in critical care and surgical emergencies in the future.

Proposed Actions

- Future studies should investigate both biological and non-biological factors contributing to disparities in ICU utilisation and post-ICU or post-surgical outcomes between men and women.
- Ensure that women's experiences are represented in healthcare systems by improving access to quality information and education on women's health.
- Encourage healthcare systems to support research on women's health and integrate evidence-based data into practice, ensuring improved decision-making regarding the risk stratification and informed consent in critical care and perioperative female patients.

References

1. ICNARC – Summary Statistics [Internet]. [cited 2023 Jun 6]. Available from: https://www.icnarc.org/Our-Audit/Audits/Cmp/Reports/Summary-Statistics
2. Mortality and global health estimates [Internet]. [cited 2023 Jun 29]. Available from: https://www.who.int/data/gho/data/themes/mortality-and-global-health-estimates
3. Raine R, Goldfrad C, Rowan K, Black N. Influence of patient gender on admission to intensive care. J Epidemiol Community Health. 1978; [Internet]. 2002 [cited 2023 Jun 29];56(6):418. Available from: /pmc/articles/PMC1732172/?report=abstract
4. Fowler RA, Sabur N, Li P, Juurlink DN, Pinto R, Hladunewich MA, et al. Sex-and age-based differences in the delivery and outcomes of critical care. CMAJ [Internet]. 2007 Dec 4 [cited 2023 Jun 29];177(12):1513–9. Available from: https://pubmed.ncbi.nlm.nih.gov/18003954/
5. Valentin A, Jordan B, Lang T, Hiesmayr M, Metnitz PGH. Gender-related differences in intensive care: A multiple-center cohort study of therapeutic interventions and outcome in critically ill patients. Crit Care Med [Internet]. 2003 Jul 1 [cited 2023 Jun

6];31(7):1901–7. Available from: https://journals.lww.com/ccmjournal/Fulltext/2003/07000/Gender_related_differences_in_intensive_care__A.2.aspx
6. Lipes J, Mardini L, Jayaraman D. Sex and mortality of hospitalized adults after admission to an intensive care unit. Am J Crit Care [Internet]. 2013 July 1 [cited 2023 Jun 6];22(4):314–319. Available from: https://doi.org/10.4037/ajcc2013225
7. Mandigers L, Termorshuizen F, de Keizer NF, Rietdijk W, Gommers D, dos Reis MD, et al. Higher 1-year mortality in women admitted to intensive care units after cardiac arrest: a nationwide overview from the Netherlands between 2010 and 2018. J Crit Care. 2021 Aug;1(64):176–83.
8. Modra L, Higgins A, Vithanage R, Abeygunawardana V, Bailey M, Bellomo R. Sex differences in illness severity and mortality among adult intensive care patients: a systematic review and meta-analysis. J Crit Care [Internet]. 2021 Oct 1 [cited 2023 Jun 6];65:116–23. Available from: https://pubmed.ncbi.nlm.nih.gov/34118502/
9. Blecha S, Zeman F, Specht S, Lydia Pfefferle A, Placek S, Karagiannidis C, et al. Invasiveness of treatment is gender dependent in intensive care: results from a retrospective analysis of 26,711 cases. Anesth Analg. 2021 June 1;132(6):1677–83.
10. Todorov A, Kaufmann F, Arslani K, Haider A, Bengs S, Goliasch G, et al. Gender differences in the provision of intensive care: a Bayesian approach. Intensive Care Med [Internet]. 2021 May 1 [cited 2023 Jun 6];47(5):577–87. Available from: https://pubmed.ncbi.nlm.nih.gov/33884452/
11. Zettersten E, Jäderling G, Larsson E, Bell M. The impact of patient sex on intensive care unit admission: a blinded randomized survey. Sci Rep. 2019;9(1):14222.
12. Larsson E, Zettersten E, Jäderling G, Ohlsson A, Bell M. The influence of gender on ICU admittance. Scand J Trauma Resusc Emerg Med. 2015 Dec;24(23):108.
13. Samuelsson C, Sjöberg F, Karlström G, Nolin T, Walther SM. Gender differences in outcome and use of resources do exist in Swedish intensive care, but to no advantage for women of premenopausal age. Crit Care. 2015;19(1):129.
14. Hill A, Ramsey C, Dodek P, Kozek J, Fransoo R, Fowler R, et al. Examining mechanisms for gender differences in admission to intensive care units. Health Serv Res [Internet]. 2020 Feb 1 [cited 2023 Jun 29];55(1):35. Available from: /pmc/articles/PMC6980949/
15. Pietropaoli AP, Glance LG, Oakes D, Fisher SG. Gender differences in mortality in patients with severe sepsis or septic shock. Gend Med. 2010 Oct;7(5):422–37.
16. Block L, Petzold M, Syrous AN, Lindqvist B, Odenstedt Hergès H, Naredi S. Age, SAPS 3 and female sex are associated with decisions to withdraw or withhold intensive care. Acta Anaesthesiol Scand. 2019 Oct;63(9):1210–5.
17. Hollinger A, Gayat E, Féliot E, Paugam-Burtz C, Fournier MC, Duranteau J, et al. Gender and survival of critically ill patients: results from the FROG-ICU study. Ann Intensive Care. 2019;9(1):43.
18. Lee M, Kang J, Jeong YJ. Risk factors for post–intensive care syndrome: a systematic review and meta-analysis. Australian Critical Care. 2020;33(3):287–94.
19. Scheunemann LP, Leland NE, Perera S, Skidmore ER, Reynolds CF, Pandharipande PP, et al. Sex disparities and functional outcomes after a critical illness. Am J Respir Crit Care Med. 2020;201(7):869–72.
20. Kim HY, Doh JH, Jang SY, Kim EK, Hahn JY, Kim DK. Gender differences in clinical profiles of stress-induced cardiomyopathy. J Cardiovasc Ultrasound [Internet]. 2017 Dec 1 [cited 2023 Aug 21];25(4):111. Available from: /pmc/articles/PMC5762693/
21. Khan NA, Daskalopoulou SS, Karp I, Eisenberg MJ, Pelletier R, Tsadok MA, et al. Sex differences in acute coronary syndrome symptom presentation in young patients. JAMA Intern Med [Internet]. 2013 Nov 11 [cited 2023 Aug 21];173(20):1863–71. Available from: https://pubmed.ncbi.nlm.nih.gov/24043208/
22. Lee P, Regenbogen S, Gawande A. How many surgical procedures will Americans experience in an average lifetime?: Evidence from three states. In: How many surgical procedures will Americans experience in an average lifetime?: Evidence from three states [Internet]. Boston:

American College of Surgeons; 2008 [cited 2023 Jun 6]. Available from: https://mcacs.org/abstracts/2008/p15.cgi
23. Surgical operations and procedures statistics - Statistics explained [Internet]. [cited 2023 Aug 21]. Available from: https://ec.europa.eu/eurostat/statistics-explained/index.php?title=Surgical_operations_and_procedures_statistics
24. Ried M, Lunz D, Kobuch R, Rupprecht L, Keyser A, Hilker M, et al. Gender's impact on outcome in coronary surgery with minimized extracorporeal circulation. Clin Res Cardiol [Internet]. 2012 Jun [cited 2023 Jun 7];101(6):437–44. Available from: https://pubmed.ncbi.nlm.nih.gov/22228145/
25. Blankstein R, Ward RP, Arnsdorf M, Jones B, Lou YB, Pine M. Female gender is an independent predictor of operative mortality after coronary artery bypass graft surgery. Circulation [Internet]. 2005 Aug 30 [cited 2023 Jun 7];112(9 SUPPL.). Available from: https://www.ahajournals.org/doi/abs/10.1161/CIRCULATIONAHA.104.525139
26. Al-Taki M, Sukkarieh HG, Hoballah JJ, Jamali SF, Habbal M, Masrouha KZ. et al. Effect of gender on postoperative morbidity and mortality outcomes: a retrospective Cohort study.
27. Grewal K, Wijeysundera D, Carroll J, Tait G. Gender differences in mortality following non-cardiovascular surgery: an observational study. [cited 2023 Jun 7]; Available from: https://www.researchgate.net/publication/51820159
28. Xu BY, Yan S, Low LL, Vasanwala FF, Low SG. Predictors of poor functional outcomes and mortality in patients with hip fracture: a systematic review. BMC Musculoskelet Disord [Internet]. 2019 Nov 27 [cited 2023 Jun 7];20(1):1–9. Available from: https://bmcmusculoskeletdisord.biomedcentral.com/articles/10.1186/s12891-019-2950-0
29. Gaudino M, Di Mauro M, Fremes SE, Di Franco A. Representation of women in randomized trials in cardiac surgery: a meta-analysis. J Am Heart Assoc [Internet]. 2021 Aug 17 [cited 2023 Jun 9];10(16):20513. Available from: https://www.ahajournals.org/doi/abs/10.1161/JAHA.120.020513
30. Hoel AW, Kayssi A, Brahmanandam S, Belkin M, Conte MS, Nguyen LL. Underrepresentation of women and ethnic minorities in vascular surgery randomized controlled trials. J Vasc Surg. 2009;50(2):349–54.
31. Rockman C, Caso V, Schneider PA. Carotid Interventions for Women: The Hazards and Benefits. Stroke [Internet]. 2022 Feb 1 [cited 2023 Jun 9];53(2):611–23. Available from: https://www.ahajournals.org/doi/abs/10.1161/STROKEAHA.121.035386
32. Bierer BE, Meloney LG, Ahmed HR, White SA. Advancing the inclusion of underrepresented women in clinical research. Cell Rep Med [Internet]. 2022 Apr 4 [cited 2023 Jun 9];3(4). Available from: /pmc/articles/PMC9043984/
33. Duma N, Aguilera JV, Paludo J, Haddox CL, Velez MG, Wang Y, et al. Representation of minorities and women in oncology clinical trials: Review of the past 14 years. J Oncol Pract. 2018;14(1):e1–10.
34. Wallis CJD, Jerath A, Coburn N, Klaassen Z, Luckenbaugh AN, Magee DE, et al. Association of surgeon-patient sex concordance with postoperative outcomes. JAMA Surg [Internet]. 2022 Feb 1 [cited 2023 Jun 6];157(2):146–56. Available from: https://jamanetwork.com/journals/jamasurgery/fullarticle/2786671
35. Statistics — Royal College of Surgeons [Internet]. [cited 2023 Jun 7]. Available from: https://www.rcseng.ac.uk/careers-in-surgery/women-in-surgery/statistics/
36. Mayhew D, Mendonca V, Murthy BVS. A review of ASA physical status - historical perspectives and modern developments. Anaesthesia [Internet]. 2019 Mar 1 [cited 2023 Aug 21];74(3):373–379. Available from: https://pubmed.ncbi.nlm.nih.gov/30648259/
37. Celik F, Edipoglu IS. Evaluation of preoperative anxiety and fear of anesthesia using APAIS score. Eur J Med Res [Internet]. 2018 Sep 11 [cited 2023 Jun 9];23(1). Available from: https://pubmed.ncbi.nlm.nih.gov/30205837/
38. Zhang Q, Guo H, Gu H, Zhao X. Gender-associated factors for frailty and their impact on hospitalization and mortality among community-dwelling older adults: a cross-sectional population-based study. PeerJ. 2018;6:e4326.

39. Analysis: women's pain is routinely underestimated, and gender stereotypes are to blame I UCL News - UCL – University College London [Internet]. [cited 2023 Jun 9]. Available from: https://www.ucl.ac.uk/news/2021/apr/analysis-womens-pain-routinely-underestimated-and-gender-stereotypes-are-blame
40. Hussain AM, Khan FA, Ahmed A, Chawla T, Azam SI. Effect of gender on pain perception and analgesic consumption in laparoscopic cholecystectomy: an observational study. J Anaesthesiol Clin Pharmacol. 2013;29(3):337–41.
41. McCarthy M. The "gender gap" in autoimmune disease. Lancet. 2000 ;356(9235):1088.
42. Schwartz JB. The influence of sex on pharmacokinetics. Clin Pharmacokinet. 2003;42(2):107–21.
43. van Eijk LT, Dorresteijn MJ, Smits P, van der Hoeven JG, Netea MG, Pickkers P. Gender differences in the innate immune response and vascular reactivity following the administration of endotoxin to human volunteers. Crit Care Med. 2007 Jun;35(6):1464–9.
44. Zellweger R, Wichmann MW, Ayala A, Stein S, DeMaso CM, Chaudry IH. Females in proestrus state maintain splenic immune functions and tolerate sepsis better than males. Crit Care Med. 1997 Jan;25(1):106–10.
45. Knöferl MW, Jarrar D, Angele MK, Ayala A, Schwacha MG, Bland KI, et al. 17 beta-Estradiol normalizes immune responses in ovariectomized females after trauma-hemorrhage. Am J Physiol Cell Physiol [Internet]. 2001; [cited 2023 Jun 29];281(4). Available from: https://pubmed.ncbi.nlm.nih.gov/11546648/
46. Klein SL. The effects of hormones on sex differences in infection: from genes to behavior. Neurosci Biobehav Rev. 2000;24(6):627–38.
47. Federman DD. The biology of human sex differences. N Engl J Med. 2006;354(14):1507–14.
48. Angele MK, Pratschke S, Hubbard WJ, Chaudry IH. Gender differences in sepsis: cardiovascular and immunological aspects. Virulence. 2014 Jan 1;5(1):12–9.
49. Bird MD, Karavitis J, Kovacs EJ. Sex differences and estrogen modulation of the cellular immune response after injury. Cell Immunol. 2008;252(1–2):57–67.
50. Miyagi M, Aoyama H, Morishita M, Iwamoto Y. Effects of sex hormones on chemotaxis of human peripheral polymorphonuclear leukocytes and monocytes. J Periodontol. 1992 Jan;63(1):28–32.
51. Reinikainen M, Niskanen M, Uusaro A, Ruokonen E. Impact of gender on treatment and outcome of ICU patients. Acta Anaesthesiol Scand. 2005 Aug;49(7):984–90.
52. Lomauro A, Aliverti A, Weatherald J, Humbert M, Riha R. Sex and gender in respiratory physiology. [cited 2023 Aug 21]; Available from: https://doi.org/10.1183/16000617.0038-2021
53. Scully EP, Haverfield J, Ursin RL, Tannenbaum C, Klein SL. Considering how biological sex impacts immune responses and COVID-19 outcomes. Nat Rev Immunol. 2020 Jul;20(7):442–7.
54. Leong HN, Earnest A, Lim HH, Chin CF, Tan CSH, Puhaindran ME, et al. SARS in Singapore--predictors of disease severity. Ann Acad Med Singap. 2006 35(5):326–331.
55. Alghamdi IG, Hussain II, Almalki SS, Alghamdi MS, Alghamdi MM, El-Sheemy MA. The pattern of Middle East respiratory syndrome coronavirus in Saudi Arabia: a descriptive epidemiological analysis of data from the Saudi Ministry of Health. Int J Gen Med. 2014;7:417–23.
56. Heffernan DS, Dossett LA, Lightfoot MA, Fremont RD, Ware LB, Sawyer RG, et al. Gender and acute respiratory distress syndrome in critically injured adults: a prospective study. J Trauma. 2011 Oct;71(4):878–83; discussion 883-5.
57. Walkey AJ, Wiener RS. Risk factors for underuse of lung-protective ventilation in acute lung injury. J Crit Care. 2012 Jun;27(3):323.e1–9.
58. Campanelli F, Landoni G, Cabrini L, Zangrillo A. Gender differences in septic intensive care unit patients. Minerva Anestesiol. 2018 Apr;84(4):504–8.
59. Sakr Y, Elia C, Mascia L, Barberis B, Cardellino S, Livigni S, et al. The influence of gender on the epidemiology of and outcome from severe sepsis. Crit Care. 2013;17(2):R50.
60. Luethi N, Bailey M, Higgins A, Howe B, Peake S, Delaney A, et al. Gender differences in mortality and quality of life after septic shock: a post-hoc analysis of the ARISE study. J Crit Care. 2020 Feb;55:177–83.

61. Wichmann MW, Inthorn D, Andress HJ, Schildberg FW. Incidence and mortality of severe sepsis in surgical intensive care patients: the influence of patient gender on disease process and outcome. Intensive Care Med. 2000 Feb;26(2):167–72.
62. Hensley MK, Bauer ME, Admon LK, Prescott HC. Incidence of maternal sepsis and sepsis-related maternal deaths in the United States. JAMA. 2019;322(9):890–2.
63. Madsen TE, Napoli AM. The DISPARITY-II study: delays to antibiotic administration in women with severe sepsis or septic shock. Acad Emerg Med. 2014;21(12):1499–502.
64. Xu J, Tong L, Yao J, Guo Z, Lui KY, Hu X, et al. Association of sex with clinical outcome in critically Ill sepsis patients: a retrospective analysis of the large clinical database MIMIC-III. Shock. 2019;52(2):146–51.
65. Desai MK, Brinton RD. Autoimmune disease in women: endocrine transition and risk across the lifespan. Front Endocrinol (Lausanne). 2019;10:265.
66. Angum F, Khan T, Kaler J, Siddiqui L, Hussain A. The prevalence of autoimmune disorders in women: a narrative review. Cureus. 2020;12(5):e8094.
67. St. Pierre SR, Peirlinck M, Kuhl E. Sex matters: a comprehensive comparison of female and male hearts. Front Physiol. 2022;22(13):831179.
68. Canto JG, Goldberg RJ, Hand MM, Bonow RO, Sopko G, Pepine CJ, et al. Symptom presentation of women with acute coronary syndromes: myth vs reality. Arch Intern Med. 2007;167(22):2405–13.
69. Mateo-Rodríguez I, Danet A, Bolívar-Muñoz J, Rosell-Ortriz F, Garcia-Mochón L, Daponte-Codina A. Gender differences, inequalities and biases in the management of Acute Coronary Syndrome. J Healthc Qual Res. 2022;37(3):169–81.
70. Desai S, Munshi A, Munshi D. Gender Bias in Cardiovascular Disease Prevention, Detection, and Management, with Specific Reference to Coronary Artery Disease. J Midlife Health [Internet]. 2021 Jan 1 [cited 2023 Aug 21];12(1):8–15. Available from: https://pubmed.ncbi.nlm.nih.gov/34188420/
71. Wenzl FA, Kraler S, Ambler G, Weston C, Herzog SA, Räber L, et al. Sex-specific evaluation and redevelopment of the GRACE score in non-ST-segment elevation acute coronary syndromes in populations from the UK and Switzerland: a multinational analysis with external cohort validation. Lancet. 2022;400(10354):744–56.
72. Xue QL. The frailty syndrome: definition and natural history. Clin Geriatr Med. 2011 Feb;27(1):1–15.
73. Burge R, Dawson-Hughes B, Solomon DH, Wong JB, King A, Tosteson A. Incidence and economic burden of osteoporosis-related fractures in the United States, 2005-2025. J Bone Miner Res. 2007 Mar;22(3):465–75.
74. Saletti-Cuesta L, Tutton L, Wright J. The relevance of gender in the care of hip fracture patients. Int J Orthop Trauma Nurs. 2016 Aug;22:3–12.
75. Carpintero P, Caeiro JR, Carpintero R, Morales A, Silva S, Mesa M. Complications of hip fractures: a review. World J Orthop. 2014;5(4):402–11.
76. Mielke MM, Vemuri P, Rocca WA. Clinical epidemiology of Alzheimer's disease: assessing sex and gender differences. Clin Epidemiol. 2014;6:37–48.
77. Kassahun WT. The effects of pre-existing dementia on surgical outcomes in emergent and nonemergent general surgical procedures: assessing differences in surgical risk with dementia. BMC Geriatr. 2018;18(1):153.
78. Soldin OP, Mattison DR. Sex differences in pharmacokinetics and pharmacodynamics. Clin Pharmacokinet. 2009;48(3):143–57.
79. Franconi F, Campesi I. Pharmacogenomics, pharmacokinetics and pharmacodynamics: interaction with biological differences between men and women. Br J Pharmacol. 2014;171(3):580–94.
80. Li K, Chen G, Hou H, Liao Q, Chen J, Bai H, et al. Analysis of sex hormones and menstruation in COVID-19 women of child-bearing age. Reprod Biomed Online. 2021;42(1):260–7.
81. Goldberg RJ, O'Donnell C, Yarzebski J, Bigelow C, Savageau J, Gore JM. Sex differences in symptom presentation associated with acute myocardial infarction: a population-based perspective. Am Heart J. 1998;136(2):189–95.

82. Chen W, Woods SL, Puntillo KA. Gender differences in symptoms associated with acute myocardial infarction: a review of the research. Heart Lung. 2005;34(4):240–7.
83. Reisner SL, Katz-Wise SL, Gordon AR, Corliss HL, Austin SB. Social epidemiology of depression and anxiety by gender identity. J Adolesc Health. 2016;59(2):203–8.
84. Government launches call for evidence to improve health and wellbeing of women in England - GOV.UK [Internet]. [cited 2023 June 29]. Available from: https://www.gov.uk/government/news/government-launches-call-for-evidence-to-improve-health-and-wellbeing-of-women-in-england
85. FitzGerald C, Hurst S. Implicit bias in healthcare professionals: a systematic review. BMC Med Ethics. 2017;18(1):19.
86. Hoffmann DE, Tarzian AJ. The girl who cried pain: a bias against women in the treatment of pain. J Law Med Ethics. 2001;29(1):13–27.
87. Sharma RK, Prigerson HG, Penedo FJ, Maciejewski PK. Male-female patient differences in the association between end-of-life discussions and receipt of intensive care near death. Cancer. 2015;121(16):2814–20.
88. Hughto JMW, Restar AJ, Wolfe HL, Gordon LK, Reisner SL, Biello KB, et al. Opioid pain medication misuse, concomitant substance misuse, and the unmet behavioral health treatment needs of transgender and gender diverse adults. Drug Alcohol Depend [Internet]. 2021;222:108674. Available from: http://ovidsp.ovid.com/ovidweb.cgi?T=JS&PAGE=reference&D=med19&NEWS=N&AN=33773869
89. Todd CM, Yu A, Lay C, Lagman-Bartolome AM. Effect of testosterone therapy on migraine frequency and disability in two transgender patients: a case report. BMJ Case Rep [Internet]. 2023;16(1) Available from: http://ovidsp.ovid.com/ovidweb.cgi?T=JS&PAGE=reference&D=medl&NEWS=N&AN=36693705
90. Samulowitz A, Gremyr I, Eriksson E, Hensing G. “Brave men” and “emotional women”: a theory-guided literature review on gender bias in health care and gendered norms towards patients with chronic pain. Pain Res Manag. 2018;2018:6358624.
91. Nandi M, Schreiber KL, Martel MO, Cornelius M, Campbell CM, Haythornthwaite JA, et al. Sex differences in negative affect and postoperative pain in patients undergoing total knee arthroplasty. Biol Sex Differ. 2019;10(1):23.
92. Bourdiol A, Legros V, Vardon-Bounes F, Rimmele T, Abraham P, Hoffmann C, et al. Prevalence and risk factors of significant persistent pain symptoms after critical care illness: a prospective multicentric study. Crit Care. 2023;27(1):199.
93. Ott J, Champagne SN, Bachani AM, Morgan R. Scoping “sex” and “gender” in rehabilitation: (mis)representations and effects. Int J Equity Health. 2022;21(1):179.
94. Chen JT, Gershengorn HB. A tale of two ICUs: one for women and one for men? Crit Care Med. 2022;50(6):1012–5.

Patient Satisfaction as an Outcome in Patient-Centred Care: Role of Diversity

7

Federico Bilotta, Katarzyna Prus, and Angelly Martinez

Key Points from the Editors

- Patient-centred care enhances satisfaction by integrating patients' values, needs, and preferences with active communication, partnership, and health promotion, leading to more personalized care.
- Gender-sensitive care, which addresses the needs of both men and women equally, is essential for fostering trust and improving satisfaction. This approach goes beyond genomics to consider patients' preferences, beliefs, religion and social context.
- LGBTQ+ patients face unique challenges and often experience disrespect or inadequate recognition from healthcare professionals. Social acceptance of their self-perceived gender and sexual orientation is crucial for improving access to care, increasing service utilization, and building trust within the healthcare system.

F. Bilotta (✉)
Department of Anesthesiology, Intensive care and pain management, "Sapienza" University of Rome, Rome, Italy

K. Prus
Department of Neurology, University Clinical Hospital No 4 - Medical University of Lublin, Lublin, Poland
e-mail: katarzyna.prus@usk4.lublin.pl

A. Martinez
Clin Ultrasound Clinical Governance Lead Organ Donation Specialist CICM SOT GCHS Intensive Care Unit, Robina, QLD, Australia
e-mail: angelly.martinez@health.qld.gov.au

V. Neskovic, F. Rubulotta (eds.), *Diversity, Gender Equity and Inclusion in Critical Care and Perioperative Medicine*,
https://doi.org/10.1007/978-3-031-86286-1_7

Main Objectives
After reading this chapter, you will be able to:

- Explain the concept of patient-centred care within a holistic framework that includes cultural, social, and religious backgrounds, as well as self-perceived gender.
- Recognize patient satisfaction as a key outcome in evaluating the quality of patient care.
- Understand the role of diversity, equity, and inclusion in patient-centred care. You will be able to discuss the reciprocal influence between patients and physicians shaped by cultural, social, religious and gender diversity and its potential influence on overall outcome.

7.1 Introduction

Patient-centred care, with a particular focus on gender diversity, is gaining increasing attention from both patients and healthcare providers. This approach emphasizes understanding patients' experiences holistically, considering aspects such as cultural, social, and religious backgrounds, as well as self-perceived gender [1, 2]. Dedicated attention to patient-centred care effectively contributes to better health outcomes, higher patient satisfaction and reduced health costs [3]. Considering the growing attention to patient satisfaction, appropriate understanding of the role of diversity in healthcare management is essential [4]. The growing importance of a holistic approach, combined with the rise of "precision medicine," which delivers more personalized care based on a patient's genomic, biochemical, and behavioural characteristics, further highlights the relevance of patient satisfaction as a key outcome in clinical research—in line with traditional measures such as morbidity, mortality, complications, and healthcare costs [5].

Diversity in patient-centred care encompasses various aspects, including race, age, gender, ethnicity, and cultural background, and should be considered not only in relation to patients but also in the healthcare workforce [6]. The aim of this chapter is to explore the importance of diversity—including gender as a qualified variable in delivering high-quality patient-centred care and improving patient satisfaction. We will define the concept of patient-centred care, examine patient satisfaction as an outcome measure of healthcare quality, and discuss the role of gender diversity in patient-centred healthcare management.

7.2 Patient-Centred Care and Patient Satisfaction as a Primary Outcome

Patient-centred care is a healthcare model that aligns with the values, needs, and preferences of patients, achieved when clinicians actively engage patients in discussions and informed decision-making about their health [7]. Hence it involves acknowledging patient perspectives on the disease, treatment and recovery. It has been reported that provision of patient-centred care may help medical personnel to understand and manage better their patient's needs. Patient-centred care should include three essential features—effective communication, partnership, and health promotion [1, 7]. When these elements are incorporated into a personalized healthcare plan based on patients' experiences and expectations, they are strongly linked to higher levels of patient satisfaction [8, 9].

Patient satisfaction is a parameter strongly associated with the concept of patient-centred care enabling to assess the extent to which the patient is content with the healthcare they received. It is one of the most important factors to determine the success of medical facility and healthcare personnel [10]. Both quantitative and qualitative evaluations of patients' experiences are essential to identify key areas for improvement, particularly where individual needs or expectations have not been fully met. Measuring patients' satisfaction should be considered as an indispensable component of the healthcare quality assessment [11]. Furthermore, there is evidence suggesting a correlation between patient experience and other health-related outcomes, particularly in relation to health equity [12]. Identifying the strengths and weaknesses of healthcare services based on the assessment of patient's requirements can become an effective tool for the formulation of public health policies [11].

How can we measure patient satisfaction, given that it is a complex, multidimensional, and often poorly defined concept? It becomes even more challenging, as this outcome is context-dependent, shaped by the subjective experiences, expectations, and preferences of each patient regarding their care [13]. Several studies aimed to provide a comprehensive overview of the factors that affect patient satisfaction level. Both patient and provider-related determinants of patients' satisfaction are reported to be significantly influenced by the gender, both patient and provider, as well as other correlating factors, such as socio-emotional behaviour, provider style of communication or perceived competence [14, 15]. Delivering high-quality medical services requires giving proper attention to diversity, both among patients and healthcare personnel.

Reflection Point Why is patient satisfaction difficult to measure accurately, and how can it be influenced by factors other than the quality of care itself? How can providers ensure that patient satisfaction is balanced with achieving the best health outcomes, without letting personal biases or expectations interfere with the actual effectiveness of treatment?

7.3 Gender Diversity in Patient-Centred Care

7.3.1 Women as Patients and Patient-Centred Care: Gender-Directed Care

The quality of care for female patients has been a long-standing issue in designing a global healthcare policy [16]. Recently, the concept of women's health has evolved, shifting from a focus solely on sexual and reproductive aspects to a broader life-course approach. The new women's health concept addresses health challenges that women share with men, but their manifestations and consequences may be more severe for female patients due to different biological and social determinants [17]. Multiple studies have highlighted that female patients are less likely to have their medical needs adequately addressed, facing poorer access to specialist care and lower levels of communication with healthcare providers [18–20]. Gender disparities can be additionally deepened by social determinants of health, which may affect the availability of medical care for women. Therefore, ensuring proper and equal access to medical services promoting women's health is essential in developing modern healthcare policies [21]..

Women's health encompasses both health risks and conditions common to both women and men, as well as those specific to women due to biological differences. Both aspects are influenced by gender, societal ideologies, and political factors. Gender-based misconceptions among healthcare providers can impact women's access to care, even for conditions they share with men. Results of recent studies reveal, that in some settings, men are more often referred to a specialist for cardiac arrhythmias, cerebral-vascular disease, vascular surgery, hip replacement, and heart transplantation [22]. Separating reproductive health services from other areas of healthcare can create challenges, such as limited access, poor coordination between care providers, and unnecessary repetition of medical services. Since women usually make more primary care visits than men, those problems may be more pronounced, especially in the presence of specific barriers such as less discretionary time, necessity for childcare or lack of resources [23].

When not addressed properly, female patients' needs and expectations may strongly affect their satisfaction with medical care. Data indicate that women rate their hospital experiences lower than men, expressing a need for more gender-sensitive nursing care, improved privacy, and better pain management [24]. It is important to note that improving patient satisfaction with medical services requires gender-sensitive care that equally addresses the needs of both men and women.

Reproductive and maternal health require sustained attention, and these aspects are essential elements of patient-centred care in female patients. The same stands for other gender-specific health issues such as breast and gynaecological cancer treatment and prophylaxis, menstrual cycle disorders, menopausal symptoms , or endometriosis [22]. Increasing medical service availability and maintaining acceptable quality of care is extremely important. At the same time assessment of women's satisfaction in this area is essential to make healthcare more responsive and culturally acceptable. While global efforts have been made to reduce maternal mortality, women's satisfaction with reproductive health and maternal care should also be addressed in developing healthcare policies. Identifying the determinants of patient satisfaction can help improve the overall patient experience. Studies report that interpersonal behaviour is one of the most important features of patient-centred care during pregnancy and childbirth. Labour and postpartum are an extremely vulnerable time for women. During this period the need for attention and care is overly important. During maternity care, women prioritize dignity and respect. Violations of their rights can create barriers to healthcare, leading to serious consequences for both mothers and newborns [25]. Dissatisfaction with medical service creates a lack of trust between women and healthcare providers, which may result in sleep disorders, post-traumatic stress disorder, fear of future vaginal delivery, decreased milk production and willingness to breastfeed, higher need for vacuum use, epidural anaesthesia, and caesarean section. It may be correlated with a lower level of neonatal care, which puts the infants at risk of higher morbidity and mortality [26]. The assessment of the mother's experience, with a strong emphasis on emotional, and psychological issues and physical safety is essential for providing high-quality delivery services [27] (Table 7.1).

Table 7.1 Determinants of patient satisfaction

Determinants of patient satisfaction in female patients	Equal access to medical services Synchronizing female reproductive services with other components of healthcare Gender-sensitive nursing care, privacy and better pain management Respectful and understanding approach during pregnancy, labour and postpartum
Determinants of patient satisfaction in LGBTQ+ patients	Inclusive approach with tolerance toward sexual orientation and gender identity Acknowledged and recognized gender-related health issues Just access to basic healthcare and gender-affirming treatment Availability of counselling and mental healthcare
Determinants of patient satisfaction related to healthcare personnel	Open attitude with emphasis on patient-centred communication Respecting patients' needs and expectations More time spent with the patient Including patients in decisions concerning diagnostic procedures and treatment plan Race, language and gender concordance between patient and provider Gender, racial, and cultural diversity in healthcare workforce

7.4 Problem of Addressing the Needs and Expectations of LGBTQ+ Patients

The lesbian, gay, bisexual, transgender, queer, and other (LGBTQ+) populations continue to face inadequate recognition in patient-centred care. [28] Given the increasing number of adolescents and adults identifying as gay, bisexual, transgender, or gender-diverse, healthcare personnel must acquire adequate knowledge of their unique medical needs. Providing tailored, specialized care that emphasizes recognizing patients' expectations can enhance health outcomes and satisfaction within this group [29].

There is a need for a culturally competent and inclusive approach to LGBTQ+ patients [30]. Unfortunately, homophobic attitudes pose a great health risk to this group causing acts of violence and discrimination and therefore limiting access to medical services. The main concern for LGBTQ+ individuals is that disclosing sexual identity to medical personnel would result in being denied appropriate medical care. Data demonstrate that the majority of LBGTQ+ patients experience a lack of courtesy and respect from healthcare professionals when utilizing medical services [31]. Social acceptance of an individual's self-perceived gender and sexual orientation is crucial for both access to and utilization of healthcare services, as well as for fostering positive relationships with medical professionals and the healthcare system [32]. It is a key element of patient-centred care for transgender and gender-nonconforming individuals and in its absence, this group experiences stigma, prejudice and discrimination. LGBTQ+ individuals face numerous barriers in access to healthcare. This strongly affects patients' experience and satisfaction with medical services. The main issues regarding this problem are based on the lack of knowledge concerning gender identity and gender-related health issues, previous negative experiences with the healthcare system or anticipation of these experiences, economic difficulties and finally situations where providers refuse to provide healthcare services to LGBTQ + patients. Gender-related discrimination may be experienced in different areas. Many individuals are denied not only gender-affirming medical interventions and mental healthcare but also primary, emergency and preventative care. Qualitative Assessment of Emergency Care Experiences Among Transgender and Gender-Nonconforming Patients [33] revealed that transgender individuals have decreased access to medical services and overall worse health outcomes in comparison to the general population. In this study, nearly half of the investigated subjects reported avoiding the emergency department when they needed emergency care. Another study reported that more than 25% of transgender patients were unable to access gender-affirming medical interventions and about half of the patients assigned female at birth were refused to obtain gynaecological care [34].

The availability of mental health-related services is an important aspect of patient-centred approach in transgender and gender-nonconforming individuals. It is reported that LGBTQ+ patients experience difficulties in accessing mental healthcare, and when it is granted, providers often demonstrate non-affirming approaches such as qualifying transgender as a form of a mental disorder [32]. Furthermore, insurers tend to deny benefits to transgender adults for routine care as well as emergency procedures when they are not aligned with the gender stated on their insurance policy, even if the procedures are medically appropriate for their current anatomy. They also refuse to cover medically necessary gender-affirming treatment [34].

Due to increasing awareness and decreasing stigma surrounding transgender individuals more patients in this group will begin to seek medical services that help to align their physical sex characteristics with their gender identity [29]. US data state that gender dysphoria may occur in up to 0.4% population [34]. It has been reported that gender affirmation treatment including hormonal therapy as well as gender-confirming surgery can significantly improve the quality of life of transgender patients.

Transgender and gender-nonconforming patients experience unwelcoming healthcare environments, with a lack of acceptance among healthcare providers and institutional barriers that limit access to both gender-affirming care and basic medical services. Gender-affirming approaches should be integrated into the healthcare process to improve the process of pursuing patient-centred care in this group. Structural interventions with comprehensive provider training programs are necessary to ensure better access to medical service, improve its utilization, and boost transgender patient experience [35]. Proper gender-sensitive care and gender affirmation policies should be incorporated into existing healthcare systems (Table 7.1).

Reflection Point Reflecting on your own experiences as a healthcare professional or patient, how can healthcare systems better integrate gender-affirming approaches into patient-centred care for transgender and gender-nonconforming individuals? Consider any barriers you've observed or encountered in accessing care. Think about how structural interventions, such as comprehensive professional training and inclusive policies, could improve both the access to and the quality of healthcare services for this group.

7.5 Healthcare Personnel Role in Patient-Centred Care

The problem of patient-centred care should be analysed from the perspective of healthcare providers. Gender is an important factor forming the relations between patients and medical personnel as well as among medical practitioners. The number of women in the healthcare workforce continues to increase [36]. At the same time, both horizontal and vertical gender segregation is still present with female practitioners reporting workplace bias from their institutions, superiors, and colleagues in the form of unfair treatment [37]. Women and minority group professionals may at the same time experience discrimination from patients such as micro-aggressions, racism or gender harassment [38]. Such attitude devalues underrepresented personnel groups and negatively influences their career trajectories, professional attainment and retention in medicine.

It has been reported that women are still underrepresented in higher-paid, procedural specialities [39]. However, there is evidence that pay disparities persist in specialities such as primary care. Female physicians generate up to 11% less visit revenue yearly than male physicians in the same practice [40]. Probably, it can be explained by the different practice styles of female physicians, which results from specific gendered expectations: patients tend to disclose more health-related information and issues to female personnel, expect more empathetic listening from them and add to the overall visit time. At the same time, the patterns of care delivery and patient interaction provided by female doctors are strongly associated with higher clinical quality metrics [41].

The data on the association between physicians' gender and patients' satisfaction are contradictory. Bertakis and Delgado [42, 43] reported a higher level of satisfaction in patients treated by female doctors in numerous research. Other data state that a positive correlation is present for other health-related outcomes such as mortality and readmission rates [44]. A cross-sectional study on physician gender impact in primary care demonstrated that patients of female doctors were more likely to receive recommended cancer screening and diabetes management, and fewer emergency room visits and hospitalizations. On the contrary, other studies report gender has no significant impact on patient satisfaction and the treatment process [45]. Considering the mixed data, the relationship between physician gender and patient experience ratings may be more pronounced in certain medical specialities.

Research results suggest that gender is still a significant factor associated with the practice styles of male and female physicians.

Women tend to work predominantly in the primary care field, paying more attention to preventive services, counselling, health education, and the psychosocial needs of their patients [36]. In quality metrics, women physicians tend to use more patient-centred communication, when compared with male doctors. This fact can be related to a specific practice, according to the idea that female personnel facilitate more open and equal communication [46]. Women tend to spend more time with patients and enable more collaborative decision-making. These features are important in the perspective of patient satisfaction ratings, but at the same time may lead to lower productivity of female physicians—if measured by the number of patients seen or resources utilized [37].

The way of communication and style of practice are the main reasons for patients to change their doctor. Data state [23] that women are more likely to do so because of dissatisfaction with provided care. The main determinants of the decision were reported as communication problems. Furthermore, female patients more often value healthcare providers who are familiar with their medical histories and prior visits, tend to discuss sensitive topics including sexual issues and domestic violence, are more open to discussion on treatment, include them in decision-making and respect their opinion. The patient-physician relationship is an important element of patient-centred care.

Evidence shows that patients are more satisfied when healthcare providers share the same cultural background such as ethnicity, language and gender. Research states that race concordance in these cases is associated with improved communication, greater treatment adherence, and higher patient satisfaction scores [47]. Language and gender compatibility have been associated with improved home medication compliance and health-related outcomes [48]. At the same time sustaining stereotypes about physicians' knowledge and capabilities based on their race and gender may limit the potential to create collaborative relationships between patients and healthcare providers [49]. Patients and physicians influence each other's opinions, attitudes, emotions, and behaviours reciprocally; therefore, cultural and gender diversity is crucial in achieving patient-centred care (Table 7.1).

7.6 Discussion

Patient satisfaction is gaining recognition as an important measure of healthcare quality. Improving patients' experience became a part of a larger endeavour to transform medical services by providing a more patient-centred approach. Pursuing patient-centred care appears as a dynamic process, where improving the responsiveness to patients' needs and including patients in decision-making should be implemented in everyday practice. Fulfilling patients' expectations requires a holistic approach, where not only physical, but also psychological, social, and spiritual aspects of wellbeing are addressed [2]. The risk of dehumanization is especially high in the modern age, where technological progress may deflect the attention of personnel away from the patients [50]. A holistic approach including gender-specific needs and gender affirmation can empower healthcare practitioners with the tools to provide optimal care, have more meaningful patient-personnel interactions, and improve health-related outcomes and quality of life [51].

Diversity in healthcare can refer to numerous qualities (Fig. 7.1). It should be addressed to both patients and medical professionals. It is hypothesized that diversity is associated with a decreased level of discrimination [52]. While it is widely believed that increasing diversity in healthcare can reduce discrimination and promote equity, achieving fair access to medical services and fostering tolerance towards minorities remains a significant challenge for both patients and healthcare professionals.

> Diversity alone does not ensure equity; therefore, more efforts are needed to decrease disparities and mitigate the impact of discrimination.

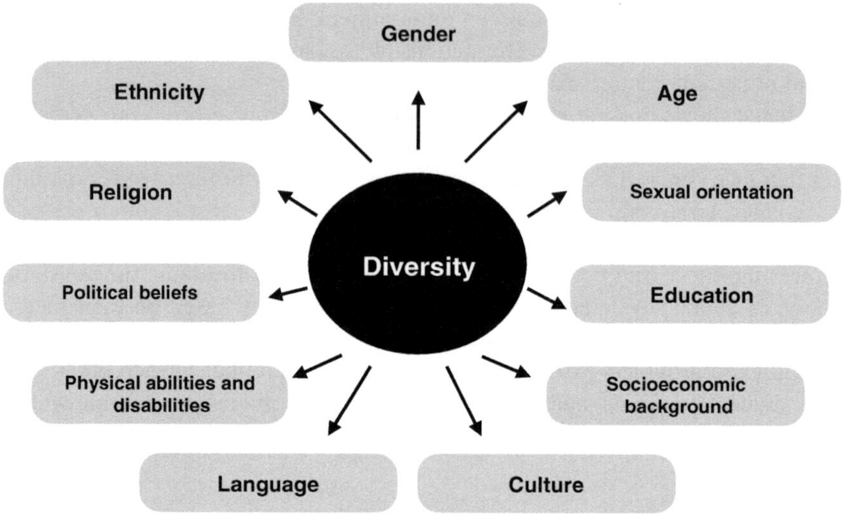

Fig. 7.1 Aspects of diversity in patient-centred care

Although increasing diversity would not eliminate all equity issues, there is sound evidence of its strong correlation with improved healthcare quality [47]. Additionally, a model of concordant care, in which patient and provider share a common attribute such as race, ethnicity, or gender is proven to improve patients' experience and satisfaction [52]. Therefore, diversity should be considered an essential element of patient-centred care and should be addressed in developing healthcare policies.

In pursuing patient-centred model of care, incorporating patients' unique gender-related needs can be an important element of precision medicine. This concept is based on incorporating a wide array of individual data, including clinical, lifestyle, genetic, and biomarker information to tailor specific treatment programs for patients. Precision medicine should not be viewed as a highly sophisticated and complex process where personalized approach to patients considers solely their genetic makeup [53]. This approach should go beyond genomics and include patients' preferences, beliefs, attitudes, and social context. Precision medicine—and the system that supports it—must embrace patient-centredness and patient engagement in the treatment process to be successful [54].

Patient satisfaction is an important tool to measure efficiency, effectiveness, and overall quality of medical services [55]. It should be considered one of the key elements of the decision-making process in healthcare management. However, qualitative and quantitative measurement of patient satisfaction is complex and challenging. The major drawback of patient satisfaction as an outcome measure results from methodology issues such as lack of psychometric standards, validation and reliability of surveys, as well as discriminatory assessment. Implementation of patient satisfaction measuring tools may be associated with potential bias due to different administrations, the acceptable response rate, the time of the survey, and the use of proxies [56]. Despite these limitations, patients' satisfaction remains an important patient-related outcome and an indicator of the quality of healthcare [13].

To conclude patient-centred care should be based not only on standard understanding of treatment management but incorporate different psychosocial and cultural aspects. Gender is an important determinant shaping the interaction between patients and healthcare providers. Diversity in this area may improve patient satisfaction levels by ensuring a better understanding of the needs, expectations, and everyday struggles of the individuals. In the patient-centred care model, patient satisfaction remains a major indicator of healthcare quality.

Proposed Actions

- Integrate patient-centred care into various medical fields, including critical care and perioperative medicine, ensuring it becomes a core component of practice.
- Incorporate patient satisfaction as a key outcome in quality-of-care assessments, alongside traditional clinical metrics such as morbidity and mortality.
- Develop curricula that emphasize diversity as a holistic approach, addressing cultural, social, religious, and gender considerations. Ensure these aspects are included in the competencies required for managing a wide range of medical conditions.

References

1. Stewart M, Belle Brown J, Weston WW, McWhinney IR, McWilliam CL, Freeman TR. Patient-centered medicine transforming the clinical method. Abingdon: Radcliffe Medical Press; 2003.
2. Mills IJ. A person-Centred approach to holistic assessment. Primary Dental J. 2017;6(3):18–23.
3. Fang C, Tanaka M. An exploration of person-centred approach in end-of-life care policies in England and Japan. BMC Palliat Care. 2022;21(1):68.
4. Getz K, Kim J. Measuring patient satisfaction as a primary outcome for patient-centric initiatives. Applied Clinical Trials. 2022;31(5)
5. Goetz LH, Schork NJ. Personalized medicine: motivation, challenges, and progress. Fertil Steril. 2018;109(6):952–63.
6. Shannon G, Jansen M, Williams K, et al. Gender equality in science, medicine, and global health: where are we at and why does it matter? Lancet. 2019;393(10171):560–9.
7. Mead N, Bower P. Patient-centredness: a conceptual framework and review of the empirical literature. Soc Sci Med. 2000;14:1087–110.
8. Little P, Everitt H, Williamson I, et al. Preferences of patients for patient centred approach to consultation in primary care: observational study. BMJ. 2001;14:468–72.
9. Han T, Li S, Li X, et al. Patient-centered care and patient satisfaction: validating the patient-professional interaction questionnaire in China. Front Public Health. 2022;10:990620.
10. Nie Y, Mao X, Cui H, et al. Hospital survey on patient safety culture in China. BMC Health Serv Res. 2013;13:228.
11. Grasso MS, Del Carmen Valls Martínez M, Ramírez-Orellana A. Health policies based on patient satisfaction: a bibliometric study. Healthcare (Basel). 2021;9(11):1520.

12. World Bank. India – equity effects of quality improvements on health service utilization and patient satisfaction in Uttar Pradesh state (English). Health, nutrition and population (HNP). Washington, DC: World Bank; 2004.
13. Ahmed F, Burt J, Roland M. Measuring patient experience: concepts and methods. Patient. 2014;7:235–41.
14. Wu CL, Naqibuddin M, Fleisher LA. Measurement of patient satisfaction as an outcome of regional anesthesia and analgesia: a systematic review. Reg Anesth Pain Med. 2001;26(3):196–208.
15. Hall JA, Roter DL, Milburn MA, Daltroy LH. Patients' health as a predictor of physician and patient behav- iour in medical visits. A synthesis of four studies. Med Care. 1996;34:1205–8.
16. Gagliardi AR, Dunn S, Foster AM, et al. Is patient-centred care for women a priority for policy-makers? Content analysis of government policies. Health Res Policy Syst. 2020;18(1):23.
17. World Health Organization. Fourth world conference on women. Geneva: WHO Press; 1995. World health organization. Women and health. Geneva: WHO Press; 2009
18. Colella TJ, Gravely S, Marzolini S, et al. Sex bias in referral of women to outpatient cardiac rehabilitation? A Meta-Analysis Eur J Prev Cardiol. 2015;22:423–41.
19. Weisz D, Gusmano MK, Rodwin VG. Gender and the treatment of heart disease in older persons in the United States, France, and England: a comparative, population-based view of a clinical phenomenon. Gend Med. 2004;1:29–40.
20. Moore JE, Mompe A, Moy E. Disparities by sex tracked in the 2015 National Healthcare Quality and disparities report: trends across national quality strategy priorities, health conditions, and access measures. Womens Health Issues. 2018;28:97–103.
21. UN.Women. Gender equality in the 2030 agenda for sustainable development: United Nations. New York: UN Women Headquarters; 2018.
22. Raine R. Does gender bias exist in the use of specialist health care? J Health Serv Res Policy. 2000;5(4):237–49.
23. Weisman CS, Rich DE, Rogers J, Crawford KG, Grayson CE, Henderson JT. Gender and patient satisfaction with primary care: tuning in to women in quality measurement. J Womens Health Gend Based Med. 2000;9(6):657–65.
24. Teunissen TAM, Rotink ME, Lagro-Janssen ALM. Gender differences in quality of care experiences during hospital stay: A contribution to patient-centered healthcare for both men and women. Patient Educ Couns. 2016;99(4):631–7.
25. Hosseini Tabar J, Shahoie R, Zaheri F, et al. Prevalence of disrespect and abuse during childbirth and its related factors in women hospitalized in the postpartum ward. J Family Med Prim Care. 2023;12(2):246–52.
26. Sacks E. Defining disrespect and abuse of newborns: a review of the evidence and an expanded typology of respectful maternity care. Reprod Health. 2017;14:66.
27. Larkin P, Begley CM, Devane D. 'Not enough people to look after you': an exploration of women's experiences of childbirth in the Republic of Ireland. Midwifery. 2012;28:98–105.
28. Uffman JC, Willer BL, Mpody C, et al. Characteristics of transgender and gender-diverse youth presenting for surgery in the United States. Anesth Analg. 2023;10
29. Lee JY, Rosenthal SM. Gender-affirming care of transgender and gender-diverse youth: current concepts. Annu Rev Med. 2023;74:107–16.
30. US Department of Health and Human Services. Advancing LGBT health and well-being. 2016. Available from: https://www.hhs.gov/sites/default/files/dhhs-lgbt-2015-annual-report.pdf?language=en
31. Klotzbaugh R, Spencer G. Lesbian, gay, bisexual, and transgender inpatient satisfaction survey: results and implications. J Patient Exp. 2020;7(1):83–8.
32. Cicero EC, Reisner SL, Silva SG, et al. Health care experiences of transgender adults: an integrated mixed research literature review. ANS Adv Nurs Sci. 2019;42(2):123–38.
33. Samuels EA, Tape C, Garber N, et al. "Sometimes you feel like the freak show": A qualitative assessment of emergency care experiences among transgender and gender-nonconforming patients. Ann Emerg Med. 2018;71(2):170–82.
34. Smith JR, Washington AZ 3rd, Morrison SD, Gottlieb LJ. Assessing patient satisfaction among transgender individuals seeking medical services. Ann Plast Surg. 2018;81(6):725–9.

35. Kearns S, Kroll T, O'Shea D, Neff K. Experiences of transgender and non-binary youth accessing gender-affirming care: a systematic review and meta-ethnography. PLoS One. 2021;16(9):e0257194.
36. Joseph MM, Ahasic AM, Clark J, Templeton K. State of women in medicine: history, challenges, and the benefits of a diverse workforce. Pediatrics. 2021;148(2):e2021051440C.
37. McMurray JE, Linzer M, Konrad TR, et al. The work lives of women physicians results from the physician work life study. The SGIM career satisfaction study group. J Gen Intern Med. 2000;15(6):372–80.
38. Solnick RE, Peyton K, Kraft-Todd G, Safdar B. Effect of physician gender and race on simulated patients' ratings and confidence in their physicians: a randomized trial. JAMA Netw Open. 2020;3(2):e1920511.
39. Rotenstein L, Gitomer R, Landon B. Pursuing gender equity by paying for what matters in primary care. N Engl J Med. 2023;10:198.
40. Ganguli I, Sheridan B, Gray J, et al. Physician work hours and the gender pay gap – evidence from primary care. N Engl J Med. 2020;383:1349–57.
41. Reid RO, Friedberg MW, Adams JL, et al. Associations between physician characteristics and quality of care. Arch Intern Med. 2010;170:1442–9.
42. Bertakis KD, Franks P, Azari R. Effects of physician gender on patient satisfaction. J Am Med Womens Assoc (1972). 2003;58(2):69–75.
43. Delgado A, Lopez-Fernandez LA, Luna JD. Influence of the doctor's gender in the satisfaction of the users. Med Care. 1993;31(9):795–800.
44. Tsugawa Y, Jena AB, Figueroa JF, Orav EJ, Blumenthal DM, Jha AK. Comparison of hospital mortality and readmission rates for medicare patients treated by male vs female physicians. JAMA Intern Med. 2017;177(2):206–13.
45. Takeshita J, Wang S, Loren AW, et al. Association of Racial/ethnic and gender concordance between patients and physicians with patient experience ratings. JAMA Netw Open. 2020;3(11):e2024583.
46. Roter DL, Hall JA, Aoki Y. Physician gender effects in medical communication: a meta-analytic review. JAMA. 2002;288(6):756–64.
47. Hilton EJ, Lunardi N, Sreedharan R, et al. Two sides of the same coin: addressing racial and gender disparities among physicians and the impact on the community they serve. Anesthesiol Clin. 2020;38(2):369–77.
48. Greenwood BN, Carnahan S, Huang L. Patient-physician gender concordance and increased mortality among female heart attack patients. Proc Natl Acad Sci USA. 2018;115(34):8569–74.
49. Schoenthaler A, Ravenell J. Understanding the patient experience through the lenses of racial/ethnic and gender patient-physician concordance. JAMA Netw Open. 2020;3(11):e2025349.
50. Secunda KE, Kruser JM. Patient-centered and family-centered Care in the Intensive Care Unit. Clin Chest Med. 2022;43(3):539–50.
51. Ventegodt S, Kande I, Ervin DA, Merrick J. Concepts of holistic care. In: Rubin IL, Merrick J, Greydanus DE, Patel DR, editors. Health care for people with intellectual and developmental disabilities across the lifespan. Springer; 2016.
52. Togioka BM, Duvivier D, Young E. Diversity and discrimination in healthcare. In: StatPearls [Internet]; 2023. Available from: https://www.ncbi.nlm.nih.gov/books/NBK568721/.
53. König IR, Fuchs O, Hansen G, von Mutius E, Kopp MV. What is precision medicine? Eur Respir J. 2017;50(4):1700391.
54. Ginsburg GS, Phillips KA. Precision medicine: from science to value. Health Aff (Millwood). 2018;37(5):694–701.
55. Jakobsson L, Holmberg L. Quality from the patient's perspective: a one-year trial. Int J Health Care Qual Assur. 2012;25:177–88.
56. Joosten EA, DeFuentes-Merillas L, De Weert G, et al. Systematic review of the effects of shared decision-making on patient satisfaction, treatment adherence and health status. Psychother Psychosom. 2008;77:219–26.

8 Cross Section of Today: Current Scenarios and Actions Taken to Promote Diversity, Equality, and Inclusivity in Patient Care

Emilio Rodriguez-Ruiz, Silvia De Rosa, and Denise Battaglini

Key Points from the Editors

- Diversity, inclusion, and equity in critical care and perioperative medicine is often hindered by subtle, implicit barriers built into the system, such as socioeconomic, religious, and cultural barriers, and societal expectations.
- National and international patient safety organizations are taking steps to promote DEI focusing on policy changes and creating a supportive environment for women and minorities.
- While data on women's outcome is available in the field of critical care and perioperative medicine, there is a lack of insight into the reasons behind their underrepresentation, which is crucial for developing effective strategies to improve equity.

E. Rodriguez-Ruiz
Intensive Care Medicine Department, University Clinic Hospital of Santiago de Compostela (CHUS), Santiago de Compostela, Spain

Simulation, Life Support, and Intensive Care Research Unit (SICRUS), Health Research Institute of Santiago de Compostela (IDIS), Santiago de Compostela, Spain
e-mail: r.ruizemilio@gmail.com

S. De Rosa
Centre for Medical Sciences-CISMed, University of Trento, Trento, Italy

Anesthesia and Intensive Care, Santa Chiara Regional Hospital, APSS, Trento, Italy

D. Battaglini (✉)
Anesthesia and Intensive Care, IRCCS Ospedale Policlinico San Martino, Genoa, Italy

V. Neskovic, F. Rubulotta (eds.), *Diversity, Gender Equity and Inclusion in Critical Care and Perioperative Medicine*,
https://doi.org/10.1007/978-3-031-86286-1_8

Main Objectives
After reading this chapter, you will be able to:

- Explain key barriers to women's care in critical care and perioperative medicine, including implicit and explicit bias.
- Explain key barriers to minorities access to provision of critical care and perioperative medicine, including implicit and explicit bias.
- Categorize international initiatives aimed at advancing DEI in healthcare, with a focus on critical care and perioperative medicine.
- Differentiate between institutional and individual efforts to raise awareness of DEI challenges and explore potential solutions.

8.1 Introduction

The principles of diversity, equality, and inclusion (DEI) are required to provide exceptional and high-quality patient care. Effective DEI practices ensure that the services provided to patients are fair and accessible to everyone and without discrimination [1]. All patients should have equal opportunities to access high-quality care and support to meet their individual needs regardless of age, race/ethnicity, gender, sexual orientation, culture, immigration status, physical disability status, or background/socioeconomic status [1]. Patient-centred care must always ensure that the unique characteristics of everyone are at the forefront of the treatment plan and that healthcare professionals are non-judgemental. A strong and comprehensive equality and diversity policy guarantees that people are treated as equals, that they get the dignity and respect they deserve, and that their differences are celebrated. Fair and equal treatment should not be viewed as an add-on to healthcare services, but as an essential right.

While enhancing DEI in healthcare may seem easy, it requires identifying barriers and biases and taking targeted actions to address the inequalities, discrimination, and marginalization experienced by certain groups of patients. Discrimination in healthcare is defined as a lack of consideration or negative actions towards an individual or a group of people because of an unjustified, preconceived opinion [2]. On the one hand, discrimination can be subtle, passive, or unintentional, such as overlooking certain things or simple stereotyping. On the other hand, discrimination can also be more overt, such as direct labelling or blatant prejudice.

Recognizing what makes people different, embracing diversity, is the first step towards equality and being aware of how some differences can impact healthcare. This chapter explores the current scenarios and international actions taken to enhance equality and diversity for patients.

8.2 Definitions of Diversity, Equality, and Inclusion in Healthcare

Diversity means appreciating the differences between people and treating people's values, beliefs, cultures, and lifestyles with respect. Within the medical field, embracing diversity means including patients, healthcare workers, trainees, educators, researchers, and people with disabilities as well as people from different social classes, socioeconomic backgrounds, racial and ethnic backgrounds, gender identities, and primary spoken languages and geographic areas. Negative acts or disregard for an individual resulting from a predetermined and unjustified view is considered as discrimination. Examples of discrimination stemming from disrespect for diversity include biases and stereotypes such as racist behaviour, discrimination against people with drug addiction, different religions, and various socioeconomic backgrounds [1].

Equality Health equality means ensuring everyone in your setting has equal opportunities for treatment, regardless of their abilities, their background, or their lifestyle. Since each subject has a different health potential, fairness in healthcare does not always include treating everyone the same or even producing "equal" results. Treatments can be more precisely tailored when variations in health and risk profiles and responsiveness to therapy between sociodemographic groups are accounted. When health potential differences cannot be attributed to biological causes, we ought to investigate the structural causes, unconscious prejudices, and other underlying causes of these differences to prevent inequity of treatment. Health inequity means that treatments are provided considering sociodemographic characteristics rather than disease's features, without evidence that this strategy results in better outcomes [1]. Inequality is not uncommon. A recent study showed that Black and Asian patients who met specific clinical thresholds for intubation and mechanical ventilation were less likely to be intubated than White patients [3]. Gender is another sociodemographic feature at risk of inequity. A study demonstrated that more men than women were admitted to intensive care units, although women were sicker than men [4]. Nevertheless, these perceived differences can vary across countries, according to sociodemographic status, religion, and geopolitical situation. A lower sickness severity was found instead in women admitted to intensive care units in Australia and New Zealand, where women were admitted to intensive care units at lower sickness severity than men [5].

Inclusion Inclusion in patient care refers to the proactive approach of ensuring that all individuals receive equitable and respectful access to healthcare services, regardless of their diverse backgrounds, characteristics, or circumstances. This means creating an environment where patients feel valued, heard, and supported and where their unique needs and perspectives are acknowledged and integrated into the care process [1]. In practice, inclusion involves actively incorporating the views and experiences of patients from various demographic groups, including those with different races, ethnicities, genders, sexual orientations, religions, cultures, socioeconomic statuses, and abilities [3]. This can also encompass individuals who may face marginalization or discrimination due to their immigration status, physical or mental health conditions, and other social determinants of health. Inclusion aims to eliminate barriers to healthcare, enhance communication and collaboration between patients and healthcare providers [5], and ensure that healthcare policies and practices uphold the principles of equity and representation. Ultimately, inclusive patient care contributes to improved health outcomes by fostering a sense of belonging and trust within the healthcare system, empowering patients to engage in their care actively.

Reflection Point
In your daily practice, are you aware of the potential barriers to delivering fair and equitable care to your patients? What weaknesses in your work environment (healthcare system, hospital, or department) could contribute to these barriers?

8.3 Current Scenarios and Challenges

Promoting DEI in healthcare has become a paramount concern. Despite the significant progress that has been made in the fight against health disparities in recent decades, much work remains to be done to fully address health inequities [6]. Table 8.1 highlights some of the current disparities in healthcare.

Achieving equality of health outcomes requires the identification of barriers and biases, and targeted action to overcome specific inequalities, discrimination, and marginalization experienced by certain groups and individuals. Below are some key challenges in achieving equality and diversity in patient care:

Healthcare Disparities or Health Inequities Inequities among different population groups can manifest as differences and/or gaps in access to care, quality of care, treatment outcomes, and overall health status [7]. Health disparities have been studied mainly based on gender, race, ethnicity, and culture. However, factors such as lifestyle choices, socioeconomic status, sexual orientation, immigration status, pri-

Table 8.1 Key examples of disparities in healthcare

Specific situations	References
US African American population has a greater burden of myocardial infarction, heart failure, stroke, and other cardiovascular events	Bonow RO, Grant AO, Jacobs AK. The cardiovascular state of the union: confronting healthcare disparities. Circulation. 2005;111(10):1205–7. https://doi.org/10.1161/01.CIR.0000160705.97642.92
Disparities secondary to gender, race and ethnicity, and geography are related to the prevalence, morbidity, and mortality associated with cardiovascular disease and its related risk factors	Mozaffarian D, Benjamin EJ, Go AS, et al. Heart disease and stroke statistics—2015 update: a report from the American Heart Association. Circulation. 2015; 131:e29–e322. https://doi.org/10.1161/CIR.0000000000000152
In the United States, minorities (Hispanics, non-Hispanic Blacks, non-Hispanic Asians and American Indians/Alaskan natives) have a higher prevalence, risk of complications, and mortality rate compared to the majority group (Non-Hispanic whites)	Centers for Disease Control and Prevention. National Diabetes Statistics Report: Estimates of Diabetes and Its Burden in the United States, 2020. US Department of Health and Human Services; Atlanta, GA: 2020
Cancer disparities are associated with multiple factors including race and ethnicity, socioeconomic status, geography, and sex. Currently, in the United States, there is a rising incidence for breast, prostate, and uterine corpus cancers, which happen to have the largest racial disparities in mortality	Siegel RL, Miller KD, Wagle NS, Jemal A. Cancer statistics, 2023. CA Cancer J Clin. 2023;73(1):17–48. https://doi.org/10.3322/caac.21763
In the United States, the incidence and prevalence of chronic kidney disease and end-stage renal disease is higher in racial and ethnic minority groups (Hispanics and non-Hispanic Blacks)	United States Renal Data System. 2023 USRDS Annual Data Report: Epidemiology of kidney disease in the United States. National Institutes of Health, National Institute of Diabetes and Digestive and Kidney Diseases, Bethesda, MD, 2023 Hall YN. Racial and ethnic disparities in end stage renal disease: access failure. Clin J Am Soc Nephrol. 2012;7(2):196–8. https://doi.org/10.2215/CJN.13021211 Patzer RE, McClellan WM. Influence of race, ethnicity and socioeconomic status on kidney disease. Nat Rev. Nephrol. 2012;8:533–41. https://doi.org/10.1038/nrneph.2012.117 Palmer Alves T, Lewis J. Racial differences in chronic kidney disease (CKD) and end-stage renal disease (ESRD) in the United States: a social and economic dilemma. Clin Nephrol. 2010;74(Suppl 1):S72–7. https://doi.org/10.5414/cnp74s072
In the United States, American Indian and Alaska Native and Black people had a shorter life expectancy at birth (65.2 and 70.8 years, respectively) compared to White people (76.4) as of 2021	Arias E, Tejada-Vera B, Kochanek KD, Ahmad FB. Provisional life expectancy estimates for 2021. Vital Statistics Rapid Release; no 23. Hyattsville, MD: National Center for Health Statistics. August 2022. https://doi.org/10.15620/cdc:118999

(continued)

Table 8.1 (continued)

Specific situations	References
Non-Hispanic Blacks/African Americans have 2.4 times the infant mortality rate as non-Hispanic Whites. Non-Hispanic Black/African American infants are almost four times as likely to die from complications related to low birthweight as compared to non-Hispanic White infants Non-Hispanic Black/African American infants had 2.9 times the sudden infant death syndrome mortality rate as non-Hispanic Whites, in 2020 In 2020, non-Hispanic Black/African American mothers were twice as likely to receive late or no prenatal care as compared to non-Hispanic White mothers	Ely DM, Driscoll AK. Infant mortality in the United States, 2021: Data from the period linked birth/infant death file. National Vital Statistics Reports; vol 72 no 11. Hyattsville, MD: National Center for Health Statistics. 2023. https://doi.org/10.15620/cdc:131356
There is a difference in reported well-being for Black and Minority Ethnic (BME) people in the United Kingdom compared to White people. This could lead to poorer physical and mental health outcomes for BME people, including lower life expectancy	Stevenson J, Rao M. Explaining levels of wellbeing in Black and Minority Ethnic populations in England. Institute for Health and Human Development. University of East London, 2014
In Australia, there is a 10-year difference in life expectancy for Aboriginal and Torres Strait Islander people	Australian Institute of Health and Welfare 2023. Aboriginal and Torres Strait Islander Health Performance Framework: summary report July 2023. Canberra: AIHW. Viewed [11/01/2024]
In Australia, 41% of Trans & Gender Diverse who needed emergency care did not attend the emergency department out of fear of being misgendered	Kerr L, Fisher CM, Jones T. TRANScending discrimination in health & cancer care: A study of trans & gender diverse Australians. La Trobe. Book, 2019. https://doi.org/10.26181/5d3e1cc21a99c
Migrant and refugee women experience poorer health outcomes, are less likely to access sexual health care, terminations, and antenatal care, are more likely to face additional challenges during the maternity period and are at a greater risk of suffering poorer child and maternal health outcomes, including mental health, compared to Australian-born women	Billet H, Vazquez Corona M, Bohren MA. Women from migrant and refugee backgrounds perceptions and experiences of the continuum of maternity care in Australia: A qualitative evidence synthesis. Women Birth. 2022;35(4):327–39. https://doi.org/10.1016/j.wombi.2021.08.005
Sex and gender differences often ignored in clinical trials which often leaves women at greater risk of side effects and poorer health outcomes	Wainer Z, Carcel C, Hickey M, et al. The Sex and Gender Sensitive Research Call to Action Group. Med J Aust. 2020; 212 (2): 57–62.e1. https://doi.org/10.5694/mja2.50426

mary spoken language, location of residence, and physical disability status can also contribute to these inequities. For example, in the United States, while overall quality in care has improved, disparities in quality and outcomes by income and race/ethnicity are large and persistent [8].

Implicit Bias It occurs when healthcare professionals have unconscious attitudes towards patients and associate stereotypes with them. It can affect healthcare professionals' decision-making processes. Thus, implicit bias may result in differential treatment and hinder the provision of equitable care, ultimately leading to poorer health care outcomes [9]. One challenge is complete and reliable information. Recognizing and addressing implicit bias is crucial in promoting diversity and equality in healthcare.

Workforce Diversity The more diverse a society becomes, the greater is the need to diversify its healthcare workforce. A successful healthcare organization provides culturally appropriate care, in a welcoming environment, to all patients. This can only be achieved by first improving inclusiveness and participation of diverse employees at all levels of the organization [10]. Evidence supports a relationship between greater workforce diversity and improved patient care, primarily through increased access for vulnerable populations and improved patient-provider interaction [11]. Concordant care, defined as a patient and provider sharing a common attribute, has been associated with improved quality of care, improved communication, longer patient visits, greater medication adherence, higher patient satisfaction scores, and improved home medication compliance and outcomes [12–15]. Such results suggest that patient-physician concordance may facilitate communication and trust.

Cultural Competence A critical skill for all healthcare professionals is to understand and respect the cultural backgrounds, values, and beliefs of their patients. Failing to do so can lead to miscommunication and mistrust. Challenges created by the shifting demographics and needs of patients can best be addressed by professionals trained in a culturally dynamic environment that supports not only increased knowledge and skills but also better care and improved access for patients [16]. Achieving cultural competence is an ongoing challenge, as it requires continuous education and training.

Affordability and Universal Access to Care Barriers to accessing health services, such as geographic location, transport, language barriers and cost, disproportionately affect marginalized populations [17]. Guaranteeing equal access to healthcare is a complex challenge that requires policy changes and solutions.

8.4 International Actions and Initiatives: Advancing Equality and Diversity in Global Healthcare

Visit World Health Organization (WHO) Health Inequality Monitor

Disaggregated data, showing how health and life outcomes differ by factors like age, economic status, and sex, is key to advancing equity. It supports policies and programmes aimed at closing gaps and promoting health for all. The Health Inequality Data Repository provides accessible datasets on various inequality topics for global audiences.

https://www.who.int/data/inequality-monitor/data

In the latest years, DEI in healthcare has evolved into a global imperative. Several international organizations are dedicated to promoting equality and diversity in healthcare on a global scale. The World Health Organization (WHO) stands as a cornerstone, advocating for health as a fundamental right and fostering international cooperation to achieve health equity [18].

The International Council of Nurses (ICN) is another crucial player, championing the cause of nursing professionals worldwide. Recognizing the role of nurses as frontline healthcare providers, the ICN advocates for gender equality, cultural competence, and inclusive policies to enhance the quality of care and patient outcomes globally [19].

While the overarching goal is universal, the strategies employed to address healthcare disparities and promote diversity vary across countries.

In the United States, for example, initiatives such as the Affordable Care Act (ACA) have sought to reduce healthcare disparities by expanding access to care and emphasizing preventive services [20]. Additionally, organizations like the Institute for Diversity and Health Equity work to eliminate healthcare disparities based on race, ethnicity, and language. In contrast, European countries often focus on social determinants of health, recognizing the impact of socioeconomic factors on healthcare access and outcomes. Initiatives such as the European Health Equity Status Report aim to monitor and address health inequalities within and between European countries [21].

The impact of international actions and initiatives on patient outcomes is evident in improved health indicators and reduced health disparities [22]. The global effort to fight against human immunodeficiency virus (HIV)/AIDS, for instance, has led to

Reflection Point

Numerous successful international initiatives have made significant progress in promoting equality and diversity in healthcare, leading to improved patient outcomes. Are you knowledgeable about any of these initiatives? If not, what do you think might be the reason for the lack of information?

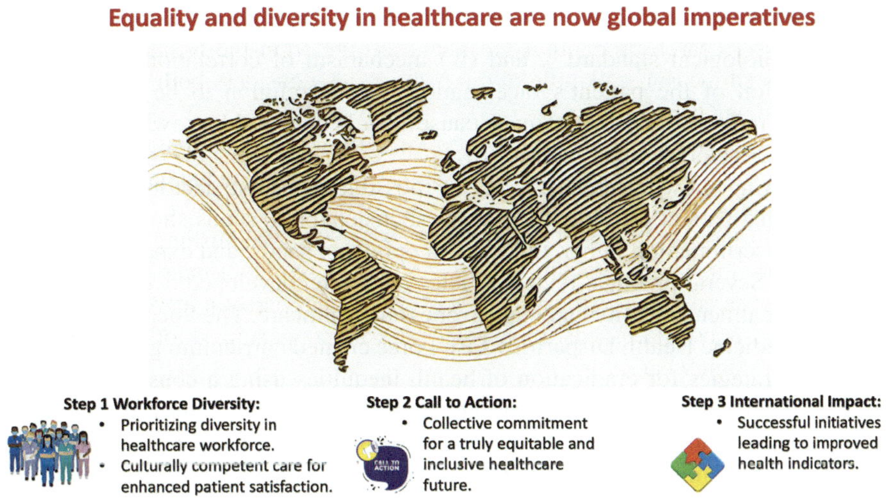

Fig. 8.1 Charting the course for global healthcare equity: a visual representation of key initiative

significant advancements in antiretroviral therapy accessibility, resulting in improved life expectancy and quality of life for affected individuals [23].

Initiatives that prioritize diversity in the healthcare workforce contribute to culturally competent care, ultimately enhancing patient satisfaction and adherence to treatment plans [24].

Despite the progress made, challenges persist in achieving global healthcare equality and diversity. Socioeconomic, cultural, and political factors continue to influence healthcare disparities. Additionally, the COVID-19 pandemic has highlighted and exacerbated existing inequities, underscoring the need for sustained international efforts.

It is imperative for nations to learn from successful initiatives, adapt strategies to their unique contexts, and collectively strive towards a world where healthcare is truly equitable and inclusive. International actions and initiatives are pivotal in advancing equality and diversity in global healthcare (Fig. 8.1). As the world continues to face evolving challenges, a commitment to DEI and collaboration remains crucial for building a healthier and more equitable future for all.

8.5 Lessons Learned and Best Practices

Education is an essential feature for achieving equality and diversity goals in healthcare. Four main mechanisms have been identified as key elements to consider for developing valid educational programmes founded on equality and diversity in healthcare, including (i) mechanism of culture (culture appears crucial in certain circumstances, worthless in others), (ii) mechanism of explicit definition of diverse culture only in those considered "strangers" (like Black people in a White people environment), (iii) mechanism of static stereotypes (variations from what is considered the "biological standard"), and (iv) mechanism of correlation or causation (consideration of the patient's race, nationality, or religion to be stated, either directly or indirectly, as the primary cause of a health problem, while in reality, other related factors were at fault [25]).

Considering these mechanisms as the possible causative factors for inequity mandates that patient's ethinicity, race, or socioeconomic status should not be the cause for discrimination rather, their health opinions, needs, and experiences really count [25]. Several practical review articles have been developed over the years to highlight treatment equality and inclusiveness in healthcare. The Society of General Internal Medicine Health Disparities Task Force created curriculum guidelines with practical strategies for eradication of health inequities using a consensus process strategy. They suggested a core curriculum focusing on three main learning objectives: (i) analyse the attitudes of patients and healthcare staff towards clinical interactions, such as mistrust, unconscious bias, and stereotyping; (ii) learn about the existence and essence of health disparities, including their multifactorial causes and the numerous challenges needed to reduce inequities; and (iii) develop the abilities to effectively communicate across different cultures, languages, and literacy levels [26]. A recent systematic review exploring the best practices for increasing education and cultural competencies against disparities found that educational programmes are currently based on interventions ranging from single-day workshops to a 10-year curriculum. The authors advised employing different instructional methodologies to increase knowledge, awareness, attitudes, and abilities. In less than half of the studies, positive results were reported. Numerous research demonstrated how challenging it is to implement curriculum without faculty members who are qualified and experienced in this topic [27]. Therefore, it is imperative to implement research and provide guidelines on the sociodemographic variations in healthcare setting, hence teaching trainers able to respond to inequity and diversity needs. Figure 8.2 represents a possible strategy to implement education and knowledge about equality and diversity in healthcare.

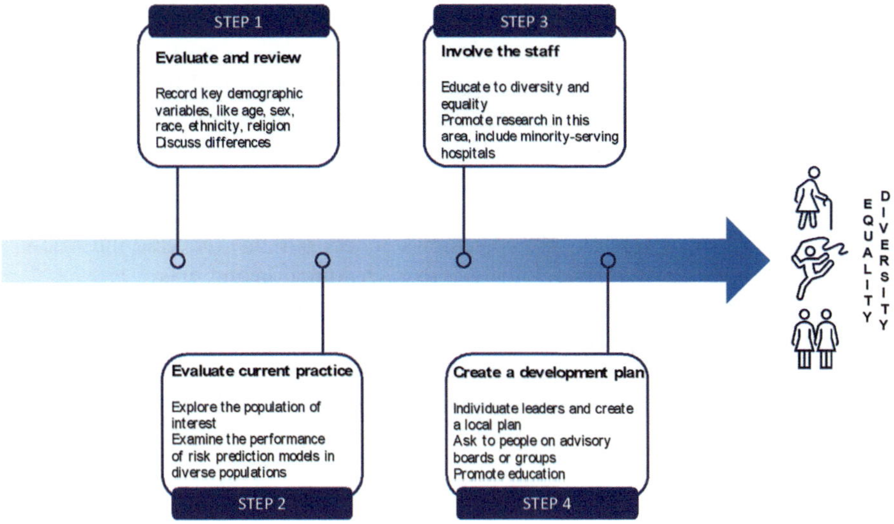

Fig. 8.2 Key steps to implement education and knowledge about equality and diversity in healthcare

8.6 Conclusions

Equality and diversity are crucial components of patient management to provide equitable and high-quality patient care. All patients should have equal opportunities to access high-quality care regardless of their unique characteristics. Currently, healthcare disparities, implicit bias, workforce diversity, cultural competence, affordability, and universal access to care are some of the key challenges in achieving equality and diversity in patient care. International actions and initiatives are pivotal in advancing equality and diversity in global healthcare. It is imperative to learn from successful initiatives, adapt strategies to each nation's unique context, and collectively strive towards a world where healthcare is truly equitable and inclusive. To guide healthcare professionals to respond to DEI needs in healthcare, future educational and research initiatives are essential.

Proposed Actions

- Foster collaboration across organizations, institutions, and individuals to drive sustainable change. Share resources, knowledge, and best practices to promote DEI in critical care and perioperative medicine. Elevate the voices of women and minorities in these fields to create lasting impact.
- Develop a system for reporting outcomes in critical care and perioperative medicine, focusing not only on sex and gender but also on other intersectional characteristics that contribute to discrimination and bias.
- Support research initiatives aimed at understanding the root causes of different outcomes based on diversity and bias.
- Promote the involvement of patients and families in decision-making, from healthcare system development to individual treatment choices.

References

1. Kotfis K, Olusanya S, Modra L. Equity in patient care in the intensive care unit. Intensive Care Med. 2024;50:291.
2. UK Public General Acts [Internet]. [cited 2024 Jan 26]. Available from: https://www.legislation.gov.uk/ukpga/2010/15/contents
3. Yarnell CJ, Johnson A, Dam T, Jonkman A, Liu K, Wunsch H, et al. Do thresholds for invasive ventilation in hypoxemic respiratory failure exist? A cohort study. Am J Respir Crit Care Med. 2023;207:271–82.
4. Todorov A, Kaufmann F, Arslani K, Haider A, Bengs S, Goliasch G, et al. Gender differences in the provision of intensive care: a Bayesian approach. Intensive Care Med. 2021;47:577–87.
5. Modra LJ, Higgins AM, Pilcher DV, Bailey MJ, Bellomo R. Sex differences in mortality of ICU patients according to diagnosis-related sex balance. Am J Respir Crit Care Med. 2022;206:1353–60.
6. Haider AH, Sexton J, Sriram N, Cooper LA, Efron DT, Swoboda S, et al. Association of unconscious race and social class bias with vignette-based clinical assessments by medical students. JAMA. 2011;306
7. Riley WJ. Health disparities: gaps in access, quality and affordability of medical care. Trans Am Clin Climatol Assoc. 2012;123:167–72.
8. Williams JS, Walker RJ, Egede LE. Achieving equity in an evolving healthcare system: opportunities and challenges. Am J Med Sci. 2016;351(1):33–43. https://doi.org/10.1016/j.amjms.2015.10.012
9. Hoffman KM, Trawalter S, Axt JR, Oliver MN. Racial bias in pain assessment and treatment recommendations, and false beliefs about biological differences between blacks and whites. Proc Natl Acad Sci. 2016;113:4296–301.
10. Kalina P. Increase inclusion to decrease physician burnout and increase wellness. J Hosp Manag Health Policy. 2019;3:18.
11. Cohen JJ, Gabriel BA, Terrell C. The case for diversity in the health care workforce. Health Aff. 2002;21:90–102.
12. Hilton EJ, Lunardi N, Sreedharan R, Goff KL, Batakji M, Rosenberger DS. Two sides of the same coin. Anesthesiol Clin. 2020;38:369–77.
13. Traylor AH, Schmittdiel JA, Uratsu CS, Mangione CM, Subramanian U. Adherence to cardiovascular disease medications: does patient-provider race/ethnicity and language concordance matter? J Gen Intern Med. 2010;25:1172–7.

14. Cooper LA, Roter DL, Johnson RL, Ford DE, Steinwachs DM, Powe NR. Patient-centered communication, ratings of care, and concordance of patient and physician race. Ann Intern Med. 2003;139:907.
15. Greenwood BN, Carnahan S, Huang L. Patient–physician gender concordance and increased mortality among female heart attack patients. Proc Natl Acad Sci. 2018;115:8569–74.
16. White KM, Zangaro G, Kepley HO, Camacho A. The health resources and services administration diversity data collection. Public Health Rep. 2014;129:51–6.
17. Williams JS, Walker RJ, Egede LE. Achieving equity in an evolving healthcare system: opportunities and challenges. Am J Med Sci. 2016;351:33–43.
18. Ruger JP, Yach D. The global role of the world health organization. Glob Health Gov. 2009;2:1–11.
19. Keighley T. Globalization, decision making and taboo in nursing. Int Nurs Rev. 2012;59:181–6.
20. Griffith K, Evans L, Bor J. The affordable care act reduced socioeconomic disparities in health care access. Health Aff. 2017;36:1503–10.
21. World Health Organization. Achieving health equity in the European region. 2019;4(10e482). https://doi.org/10.1016/S2468-2667(19)30181-1
22. Bombard Y, Baker GR, Orlando E, Fancott C, Bhatia P, Casalino S, et al. Engaging patients to improve quality of care: a systematic review. Implement Sci. 2018;13:98.
23. Kumah E, Boakye DS, Boateng R, Agyei E. Advancing the global fight against HIV/aids: strategies, barriers, and the road to eradication. Ann Glob Health. 2023;89:83.
24. Stanford FC. The importance of diversity and inclusion in the healthcare workforce. J Natl Med Assoc. 2020;112:247–9.
25. Zanting A, Meershoek A, Frambach JM, Krumeich A. The 'exotic other' in medical curricula: rethinking cultural diversity in course manuals. Med Teach. 2020;42:791–8.
26. Smith WR, Betancourt JR, Wynia MK, Bussey-Jones J, Stone VE, Phillips CO, et al. Recommendations for teaching about racial and ethnic disparities in health and health care. Ann Intern Med. 2007;147:654.
27. Brottman MR, Char DM, Hattori RA, Heeb R, Taff SD. Toward cultural competency in health care: a scoping review of the diversity and inclusion education literature. Acad Med. 2020;95:803–13.

Part III

Health Care Providers: Improving Working Environment to Gender Equity and Diversity

9 Gap and Underrepresentation of Gender and Minorities in Critical Care and Perioperative Medicine

Joana Berger-Estilita, Fiona Melanie, and Marko Zdravkovic

Key Points from the Editors

- The underrepresentation of gender and minorities in perioperative and critical care medicine is rooted in a historically privileged male-dominated environment, and it is still resistant to change.
- Many institutions and organizations are beginning to recognize the importance and the negative impact of underrepresentation of gender and minorities and are implementing strategies to address it. However, the effectiveness and sustainability of these strategies remain inconsistent.

Supplementary Information The online version contains supplementary material available at https://doi.org/10.1007/978-3-031-86286-1_9.

J. Berger-Estilita (✉)
FMH für Anästhesiologie und Intensivmedizin, Consultant in Anaesthesiology and Intensive Care Salemspital, Hirslanden Medical Group, Bern, Switzerland

Institute for Medical Education, University of Bern, Bern, Switzerland

F. Melanie
Uhor, University of Bern, Bern, Switzerland

Faculty of Medicine, University of Ljubljana, Ljubljana, Slovenia
e-mail: fiona.uhor@students.unibe.ch

M. Zdravkovic
Faculty of Medicine, University of Maribor, Maribor, Slovenia

Department of Anesthesiology, Intensive Care and Pain Management, University Medical Centre Maribor, Maribor, Slovenia

V. Neskovic, F. Rubulotta (eds.), *Diversity, Gender Equity and Inclusion in Critical Care and Perioperative Medicine*,
https://doi.org/10.1007/978-3-031-86286-1_9

- Monitoring and reporting demographic changes and the effectiveness of applied measures are essential for success. This approach acts as a diagnostic tool, identifying weaknesses and areas for further improvement.

Main Objectives

After reading this chapter, you will be able to:

- Describe existing forms of underrepresentation of gender and minorities within the perioperative and critical care environment.
- Recognize factors that contribute to perpetuating underrepresentation of these groups.
- Evaluate the effectiveness of current strategies aimed at promoting equity and inclusion.

9.1 Introduction

The underrepresentation of gender and minorities in critical care and perioperative medicine is a persistent and concerning problem in healthcare. Despite advancements in gender equality and diversity initiatives, women and minority individuals continue to face considerable barriers and challenges in pursuing careers in these specialized areas of medicine [1, 2]. This gap in representation has far-reaching implications for both healthcare providers and patients.

Historically, medicine has been dominated by a male-centric culture, with limited opportunities for women and minorities to excel in the profession as a whole [3]. The lack of diversity within our fields, namely critical care and perioperative medicine, perpetuates biases and stereotypes, affecting patient care, research outcomes, and overall healthcare quality [4, 5]. Furthermore, the underrepresentation of diverse perspectives hinders innovation and limits the profession's ability to address the needs of a diverse patient population effectively [6].

This chapter aims to shed light on the gap and underrepresentation of gender and minorities in critical care and perioperative medicine. By examining the historical context, societal and institutional factors, and the impact of underrepresentation, this chapter aims to highlight the significance of this issue within the healthcare field.

Furthermore, it seeks to emphasize the need for increased diversity and inclusion in critical care and perioperative medicine. By providing a comprehensive understanding of the barriers and challenges faced by gender and minority individuals, we aim to advocate for change and prompt discussions on strategies to address the underrepresentation and promote equal and equitable opportunities.

Ultimately, we aim to inspire action and foster a more inclusive and equitable future in critical care and perioperative medicine. By recognizing the importance of diversity, we can work towards dismantling the barriers that hinder the full participation and contribution of gender and minority individuals, thereby improving healthcare outcomes for all patients.

9.2 Historical Context and Current State

The underrepresentation of gender and minority groups in medicine is deeply rooted in history. Traditionally, medicine was predominantly male-dominated, with women and minorities facing significant barriers to entry. Gender disparities date back centuries, with women excluded from formal medical education and denied the opportunity to practice medicine. Similarly, minority individuals, particularly people of colour and foreigners, faced systemic discrimination and exclusion [7].

The nineteenth century saw some progress in gender diversity, with the first female physicians and surgeons breaking barriers in the United States and Europe. Elizabeth Blackwell, who earned her medical degree in 1849, became the first woman to receive a medical degree in the United States [8]. Despite these early trailblazers, gender and racial disparities persisted throughout the twentieth century.

In contemporary critical care and perioperative medicine, the persistent underrepresentation of both gender and minority groups remains a critical concern. Statistical data underscores the gravity of this issue, shedding light on the extent of the gap that exists in these fields [1, 9].

Women continue to face significant underrepresentation in critical care and perioperative specialities. The proportion of female intensivists and perioperative physicians significantly lags behind their male counterparts. While specific numbers may vary by region and country, it's essential to provide examples to illustrate the extent of underrepresentation:

- In many countries, women make up less than 30% of intensivists and perioperative physicians, highlighting a significant gender gap within these specialities [10].
- Women represent a minority among leadership positions in acute care, with only 15% serving as department heads or in other key leadership roles [11].
- Women appear less driven to achieve leadership positions in acute care compared to men [9].
- Women are more likely to experience mistreatment in the workplace compared to men [12].

- The underrepresentation of women in these specialities becomes even more pronounced when considering women of colour, who may represent less than 10% of the workforce in some regions [13].

On the other hand, in Europe, there is evident improvement in the proportion of women in perioperative medicine (ranging from 34% to 71%) to the extent that in at least 23 European countries women represent the majority of clinicians in our fields [14]. However, this higher proportion of women is only slowly reflected also in their inclusion in leadership positions and research opportunities, but the trend is certainly positive [9, 15].

These numbers emphasize the gravity of the underrepresentation issue in critical care and perioperative medicine, demonstrating the need for comprehensive strategies to address the gender gap and promote diversity in these disciplines. Gender gap is not limited to a specific region but is a global concern, reflecting the need for broader initiatives to promote gender diversity within these medical disciplines [1, 2].

Racial and ethnic minority groups, in particular, experience substantial underrepresentation in critical care and perioperative medicine. This challenge is particularly pronounced in countries with diverse populations, where disparities in healthcare access and career opportunities persist [7, 16]. Minority individuals often encounter additional barriers that hinder their entry and advancement in these medical specialities.

The experiences of individuals with intersecting identities, such as women of colour, further amplify the hurdles they face in critical care and perioperative medicine. The intersection of gender and racial identity compounds the challenges of underrepresentation and discrimination, highlighting the need for a more inclusive and equitable approach to address these disparities [2, 17]. Recognizing the intersectionality of identities is essential for implementing effective strategies to promote diversity and inclusivity in these fields [18].

9.3 Factors Contributing to the Gap and Underrepresentation

Several factors contribute to the persistent gap and underrepresentation in critical care and perioperative medicine.

- Implicit biases, often unconscious, influence decision-making and perpetuate stereotypes [3, 19]. These biases affect the recruitment and advancement of gender and minority individuals in medical specialities.
- Societal norms and expectations shape career choices and discourage women and minorities from pursuing critical care and perioperative medicine. Cultural expectations and stereotypes can deter individuals from entering these fields [17, 18].
- Structural challenges in medical education and training programs limit diversity in the healthcare workforce. Admissions processes, curriculum design, and men-

torship opportunities can inadvertently exclude gender and minority individuals [20].
- The absence of diverse role models and mentors in critical care and perioperative specialities hinders career development, with a lack of representation perpetuating the underrepresentation cycle [21, 22].

Reflection Point Consider the impact of the absence of diverse role models and mentors in perioperative and critical care specialties. How might the lack of representation affect career development and career trajectories? What steps can be taken to foster inclusive mentorship opportunities and ensure individuals from all backgrounds feel encouraged to pursue career in these specialties? Can you reflect on your personal experience?

Pregnancy if you wish to learn more about work condition during pregnancy in perioperative medicine, please watch this short video.

VIDEO LEGEND: "In her lecture, Dr. Joana Berger Estilita addresses the gender situation in Europe with a 2023 update, presented at the seventh edition of the World Day of Critical Lung. She explores the significance of gender parity and the persistent issue of gender bias and presents survey results on work conditions during pregnancy across European countries."

9.4 Understanding the Impact of Underrepresentation

The consequences of underrepresenting gender and minority individuals in critical care and perioperative medicine extend far beyond the confines of the healthcare profession. These repercussions are acutely felt in patient care and healthcare outcomes, where the impact is substantial. Patients from underrepresented groups often experience lower trust and communication with healthcare providers who do not share their backgrounds or experiences [23, 24]. Such disparities in trust and communication can culminate in suboptimal healthcare experiences and, consequently, compromised healthcare outcomes. Bridging this gap in representation is fundamental to fostering trust and effective communication within healthcare settings.

Underrepresentation also significantly contributes to healthcare disparities, with minority patients enduring unequal access to specialized care and, in some instances, encountering worse health outcomes [16, 25]. These disparities not only affect individual patients but also perpetuate systemic inequities within healthcare systems [26].

In addition, the limited diversity among researchers in these fields often results in significant research gaps, with critical questions and diverse perspectives going unexplored [5, 27]. Research encompassing various backgrounds and experiences leads to more comprehensive and innovative studies that can yield valuable insights [28]. Promoting diversity within research teams is pivotal in addressing these research gaps and advancing medical knowledge.

Moreover, gender and minority individuals encounter unique hurdles on their path to career advancement [13]. These hurdles include biases at various career stages, the need for more mentorship opportunities, and limited networking prospects.

In addition, the cumulative effects of bias and underrepresentation can exact a toll on healthcare professionals' psychological well-being. The stressors of navigating these obstacles can lead to burnout, diminished job satisfaction, and reduced overall well-being [29]. Recognizing and addressing the psychological toll of underrepresentation is imperative in fostering a supportive and nurturing environment for healthcare providers.

Reflection Point Healthcare professionals' well-being should be a key component of sustainability policies. How might challenges such as bias, stereotypes, and the "glass ceiling" impact job satisfaction, stress levels, and overall well-being? What strategies or changes within healthcare environments could help alleviate these pressures? Have you observed any positive changes in your own work environment?

9.5 Sociocultural Factors Fostering Underrepresentation

The landscape of critical care and perioperative medicine is intricately entwined with sociocultural factors perpetuating stereotypes and biases. Stereotypes regarding the capabilities and suitability of individuals based on their gender or minority status have long plagued these medical fields. Both explicit and implicit biases affect perceptions of competence and suitability, influencing decisions related to recruitment, promotion, and career advancement.

Sociocultural norms and societal expectations regarding gender roles and career choices can significantly influence individuals' decisions in career choices. Gender-specific expectations may deter women from pursuing roles in critical care and perioperative medicine, while cultural pressures can constrain career choices for minorities. Additionally, healthcare providers may unknowingly harbour implicit biases influencing patient care decisions. These biases can result in differential treatment, misdiagnoses, and suboptimal care for patients from gender and minority groups [30].

9.6 Institutional Factors

Medical education and training programs often contain structural barriers that inadvertently hinder diversity and perpetuate underrepresentation. There is a significant gap in mentorship opportunities for underrepresented individuals, which can preclude career progression and limit access to valuable guidance [31]. Building professional networks is vital in any field, but gender and minority individuals may face challenges in networking due to less diverse existing networks. Creating inclusive networking opportunities can level the playing field. It is important to establish formal mentorship programs specifically designed to support gender and minority individuals [31]. Structured guidance and support programs play a critical role in helping individuals navigate the complexities of critical care and perioperative medicine. However, institutional policies and practices may unintentionally perpetuate underrepresentation. For example, promotion criteria often fail to adequately recognize diverse contributions or account for the unique challenges faced by women and minority groups. This highlights the need to reevaluate these criteria to ensure fairness and inclusivity.

While many institutions have implemented diversity initiatives, their impact can vary significantly. To move beyond symbolic gestures, these initiatives must translate into tangible change. Holding institutions accountable is essential, including ensuring transparency in reporting diversity data and setting measurable goals. Such actions can drive meaningful progress toward a more equitable and inclusive professional environment.

9.7 Strategies for Addressing the Gap

To address the underrepresentation of gender and minority individuals in critical care and perioperative medicine, a proactive approach ***begins with promoting diversity and inclusion in medical education and training.***

- Medical schools and training programs can reassess their admissions processes to ensure they do not inadvertently disadvantage gender and minority applicants. Implementing holistic admissions criteria that consider applicants' diverse backgrounds and experiences can contribute to a more equitable selection process.
- Medical curricula should be updated to incorporate a more inclusive approach integrating topics related to gender and minority health, cultural competency training, and exposure to diverse patient populations. By fostering an environment that values diversity from the outset, medical education can better prepare future healthcare professionals to serve a diverse patient base.
- Education and training programs should prioritize cultural competency training to equip healthcare providers with the skills needed to understand and address

the unique needs of patients from different backgrounds. This training should encompass not only clinical skills but also effective communication and empathy.

- Institutions and professional organizations should establish formal mentorship programs tailored to the needs of gender and minority individuals. These programs can pair early-career professionals with experienced mentors who can provide guidance, career advice, and emotional support.
- Encouraging diversity in leadership positions within medical organizations and departments can create more inclusive environments. When individuals see leaders who reflect their own backgrounds, it can inspire confidence and ambition in pursuing leadership roles.
- Institutions should establish confidential and safe reporting mechanisms for incidents of discrimination, harassment, or bias. Creating an environment where individuals can report such incidents without fear of retaliation is crucial for fostering inclusivity.
- Medical institutions should regularly review and revise their promotion criteria to ensure they recognize diverse contributions and experiences. Creating transparent and inclusive promotion pathways can help individuals from underrepresented groups advance in their careers.
- Appointing diversity and inclusion officers within medical organizations can provide dedicated leadership in driving diversity efforts. These officers can work on implementing and monitoring diversity initiatives and holding institutions accountable for their progress.
- Institutions should collect and report demographic data to assess their progress towards diversity and inclusion goals. Transparency in reporting can shed light on areas that require improvement and drive the adoption of more inclusive policies.

9.8 Future Directions and Recommendations

As we look towards the future, it is imperative to promote research focused on gender and minority representation in critical care and perioperative medicine. Comprehensive studies should investigate the impact of diversity on patient outcomes, the effectiveness of diversity initiatives, and the experiences of underrepresented individuals in these fields. Research findings can ***inform evidence-based strategies*** to enhance diversity and inclusion.

Addressing the underrepresentation of gender and minority individuals requires collaborative efforts and partnerships. Medical organizations, academic institutions, professional societies, and policymakers must come together to share best practices, develop joint initiatives, and advocate for systemic change. By pooling resources and expertise, these collaborative efforts can drive meaningful progress.

Sustainability is the key to ensuring lasting diversity and inclusion. Long-term strategies should focus on integrating diversity principles into the core values of medical institutions. This includes ongoing education, mentorship programs, accountability measures, and continuous monitoring of progress. By making diversity and inclusion an integral part of the medical landscape, we can create a future where underrepresentation is no longer a barrier.

9.9 Conclusion

The underrepresentation of gender and minority individuals in critical care and perioperative medicine is a complex issue deeply rooted in history. However, by understanding the historical context, acknowledging the current situation, and recognizing the multifaceted factors contributing to the gap, we can pave the way for change. In several countries, there is a positive trend in this direction which must be continued. The impact of underrepresentation on patients, healthcare outcomes, research, and career advancement underscores the urgency of addressing this issue.

This chapter has outlined strategies to bridge the gap, including promoting diversity and inclusion in education, creating supportive environments, advocating for policy changes, and fostering research and partnerships. It is a call to action for individuals, institutions, and policymakers to collectively work towards a more inclusive and equitable future in critical care and perioperative medicine. While challenges remain, there is hope that through concerted efforts and a commitment to diversity, we can achieve a healthcare landscape that truly reflects the rich tapestry of our society and ensures that every voice is heard and valued.

Action Points

- Determine zero tolerance to discrimination and harassment. Establish a confidential and safe policy for reporting and addressing incidents of discrimination, harassment, or bias in medical faculties, hospitals, and departments.
- Appoint diversity and inclusion officers within medical organizations to provide dedicated leadership and drive of diversity initiatives.
- Monitor and regularly publish reports on demographic changes to track progress and ensure the sustainability of positive changes over time.

At the following link, find the presentation on the reasonsfor individual and systemic need to develop **Gender Equity Plans**.

VIDEO LEGEND: "Sarah Saxena presents at the World Day of Critical Lung, outlining the need for both individual and systemic approaches to developing a comprehensive Gender Equity Plan."

References

1. Bosco L, Lorello GR, Flexman AM, Hastie MJ. Women in anaesthesia: a scoping review. Br J Anaesth. 2020;124(3):e134–e47.
2. Gisselbaek M, Barreto Chang OL, Saxena S. Gender equity in anesthesia: is it time to rock the boat? BMC Anesthesiol. 2023;23(1):67.
3. Noronha B, Fuchs A, Zdravkovic M, Berger-Estilita J. Gender balance in the medical workplace—A snapshot into anesthesia. Tren Anaesth Crit Care. 2022;43:4–10.
4. Hawkes S, Haseen F, Aounallah-Skhiri H. Measurement and meaning: reporting sex in health research. Lancet. 2019;393(10171):497–9.
5. Petkovic J, Trawin J, Dewidar O, Yoganathan M, Tugwell P, Welch V. Sex/gender reporting and analysis in Campbell and Cochrane systematic reviews: a cross-sectional methods study. Syst Rev. 2018;7(1):113.
6. Stanford FC. The importance of diversity and inclusion in the healthcare workforce. J Natl Med Assoc. 2020;112(3):247–9.
7. Banaji MR, Fiske ST, Massey DS. Systemic racism: individuals and interactions, institutions and society. Cogn Res: Prin Implic. 2021;6(1):82.
8. Bristol Uo. Who was Elizabeth Blackwell? 2023. Available from: https://www.bristol.ac.uk/blackwell/what-we-do/who-was-elizabeth-blackwell/.
9. Zdravkovic M, Osinova D, Brull SJ, Prielipp RC, Simões CM, Berger-Estilita J. Perceptions of gender equity in departmental leadership, research opportunities, and clinical work attitudes: an international survey of 11 781 anaesthesiologists. Br J Anaesth. 2020;124(3):e160–e70.
10. Venkatesh B, Mehta S, Angus DC, Finfer S, Machado FR, Marshall J, et al. Women in Intensive Care study: a preliminary assessment of international data on female representation in the ICU physician workforce, leadership and academic positions. Crit Care. 2018;22(1):211.
11. Mose JN. Representation of Women in Top Executive Positions in General Medical-Surgical Hospitals in the United States. Womens Health Rep (New Rochelle). 2021;2(1):124–32.
12. Berger-Estilita J, Fritsche L, El-Boghdadly K, Dias CC, Zdravkovic M. European anesthesiologists' experiences with gender-based mistreatment in the workplace: a secondary multilevel regression analysis. Korean J Anesthesiol. 2024;77(1):46–57.
13. Pogrebna G, Angelopoulos S, Motsi-Omoijiade I, Kharlamov A, Tkachenko N. The impact of intersectional racial and gender biases on minority female leadership over two centuries. Sci Rep. 2024;14(1):111.
14. Eurostat. Majority of health jobs held by women 2021 2021. Available from: https://ec.europa.eu/eurostat/web/products-eurostat-news/-/edn-20210308-1.
15. Basile ER, Byrd H, Powell-Williams M, Polania Gutierrez JJ, Riveros-Perez E. Gender gap: a qualitative study of women and leadership acquisition in anesthesiology. Anesth Analg. 2023;136(1):6–12.
16. Khusid E, Lui B, Ibarra A, Villegas K, White RS. Review of racial/ethnic disparities in obstetrics-related anesthesia administration and pain management. Pain Manag. 2023;13(7):415–22.
17. Coe IR, Wiley R, Bekker LG. Organisational best practices towards gender equality in science and medicine. Lancet. 2019;393(10171):587–93.
18. Hooks B. Feminism is for everybody: passionate politics. South End Press; 2000.
19. Witteman HO, Hendricks M, Straus S, Tannenbaum C. Are gender gaps due to evaluations of the applicant or the science? A natural experiment at a national funding agency. Lancet. 2019;393(10171):531–40.
20. Gause SA, Vranas KC. Workforce diversity and equity among critical care physicians. Crit Care Clin. 2024;40(4):767–87.
21. Healy NA, Cantillon P, Malone C, Kerin MJ. Role models and mentors in surgery. Am J Surg. 2012;204(2):256–61.
22. Flexman AM, Gelb AW. Mentorship in anesthesia. Curr Opin Anesthesiol. 2011;24(6):676.
23. Bazargan M, Cobb S, Assari S. Discrimination and medical Mistrust in a racially and ethnically diverse sample of california adults. Ann Fam Med. 2021;19(1):4–15.

24. Moore C, Coates E, Watson A, de Heer R, McLeod A, Prudhomme A. "It's important to work with people that look like me": black patients' preferences for patient-provider race concordance. J Racial Ethn Health Disparities. 2023;10(5):2552–64.
25. Williams DR, Rucker TD. Understanding and addressing racial disparities in health care. Health Care Financ Rev. 2000;21(4):75–90.
26. Gutiérrez Gutiérrez J, Carrasco González MD, Montiel González R, San Barón M, Barea Mendoza JA, Giménez-Esparza Vich C, et al. Challenges in intensive medicine: diversity, equity and inclusion. Gender statement of the Spanish Society of Intensive and Critical Medicine and Coronary Units (SEMICYUC). Med Intensiva (Engl Ed). 2023;47(7):402–5.
27. Antequera A, Cuadrado-Conde MA, Roy-Vallejo E, Montoya-Martínez M, León-García M, Madrid-Pascual O, et al. Lack of sex-related analysis and reporting in Cochrane reviews: a cross-sectional study. Syst Rev. 2022;11(1):281.
28. Turi JA, Khastoori S, Sorooshian S, Campbell N. Diversity impact on organizational performance: moderating and mediating role of diversity beliefs and leadership expertise. PLoS One. 2022;17(7):e0270813.
29. Rhead RD, Chui Z, Bakolis I, Gazard B, Harwood H, MacCrimmon S, et al. Impact of workplace discrimination and harassment among National Health Service staff working in London trusts: results from the TIDES study. BJPsych Open. 2020;7(1):e10.
30. Hall WJ, Chapman MV, Lee KM, Merino YM, Thomas TW, Payne BK, et al. Implicit racial/ethnic bias among health care professionals and its influence on health care outcomes: a systematic review. Am J Public Health. 2015;105(12):e60–76.
31. Edwards KJ, Akam E, Ijoma JN, Mack KN, Pereira PMR, Dhanvantari S, et al. Visions by WIMIN: global mentorship to retain underrepresented trainees. Mol Imaging Biol. 2022;24(4):519–25.

Diversity, Equity, and Inclusion: Key Changes Needed: Essential, Recommended, and Optional

10

Cristina Santonocito, Madiha Hashmi, Filippo Sanfilippo, Aasma Khan, Maham Jawaid Ahmad, Luigi La Via, Luciana Mascia, and Francesca Rubulotta

Supplementary Information The online version contains supplementary material available at https://doi.org/10.1007/978-3-031-86286-1_10.

C. Santonocito
Department of Anesthesia and Intensive Care – CAST Rodolico San Marco University Hospital, Catania, Italy

M. Hashmi
Department of Critical Care Medicine, Ziauddin University, Karachi, Pakistan

CCM Fellowship & MD Programme, Ziauddin Group of Hospitals, Visiting Faculty, Aga Khan University, Karachi, Pakistan

Honorary Physician MORU, Bangkok, Secretary Faculty of CCM, Bangkok, Thailand

F. Sanfilippo
Department of Anesthesia and Intensive care – Policlinico Rodolico San Marco University hospital Catania, Catania, CT, Italy

A. Khan · M. J. Ahmad
Department of Critical Care Medicine, Ziauddin University, Karachi, Pakistan
e-mail: aasma.khan@zu.edu.pk

L. L. Via
Department of Anesthesia and Intensive Care, University Hospital Policlinico G. Rodolico-San Marco, Catania, Italy
e-mail: luciana.mascia@unisalento.it

L. Mascia
Dipartimento di Medicina Sperimentale, University of Salento, Lecce, Italy
e-mail: luciana.mascia@unisalento.it

F. Rubulotta (✉)
Department of Anaesthesia and Critical Care, Ospedale Gaspare Rodolico, Catania, Italy

International Women in Intensive and Critical Care Medicine, iWIN ETS, Catania, Italy
e-mail: francesca.rubulotta@unict.it

V. Neskovic, F. Rubulotta (eds.), *Diversity, Gender Equity and Inclusion in Critical Care and Perioperative Medicine*,
https://doi.org/10.1007/978-3-031-86286-1_10

Key Points from the Editors

- It is essential to identify the actions needed to support DEI and categorize them into essential, recommended, and optional to prioritize initiatives and allocate often limited resources effectively. Creating such a list also helps assess the current state of the institution and provides a framework for benchmarking progress.
- Sponsorship and mentorship are encouraged from early stages of career to generate a culture of support and team building.
- Childcare is part of individual work-life balance. Facilities to support healthcare workers parenting will improve performance and ultimately patients' care.

Main Objectives

After reading this chapter, you will be able to:

- Identify key areas for improving diversity, equity, and inclusion (DEI) within healthcare.
- Evaluate actions—essential, recommended, or optional—needed to reduce the gender gap and promote DEI, and understand how these actions can contribute to improved women leadership.
- Recognize the differing priorities for DEI in healthcare across countries of varying income levels (high, upper-middle, lower-middle, and low-income).

10.1 Introduction

Healthcare studies showed patients improved when heterogeneous teams provided care [1]. Diversity, gender equity, and inclusion (DEI) in a team bring heterogeneity in thoughts, skills, and potentially better outcomes for the patients [1]. Professional skills-focused studies generally find improvements to innovation, team communication, and improved risk assessment [1]. Increased diversity has been linked to improved financial performance, suggesting that a diversity-friendly environment helps reduce the challenges and resistance typically associated with organizational change [1].

Over the past few decades, there has been a gradual increase in the representation of women, LGBT+, and minority groups in the medical profession. However, these groups remain underrepresented in leadership positions [2]. In 2013, the issue of inequality in healthcare and career progression gained significant attention [3]. One key approach to improving the working lives of physicians is to ensure that healthcare systems are genuinely inclusive [4]. An independent study, 'Fair to Refer?', revealed that some individuals still face marginalization and remain in 'outsider' groups within healthcare organizations [5]. Addressing these issues of inclusion is essential not only to retain doctors but also to enable them to perform at their best. Compassionate and inclusive leadership is critical for both the well-being of the workforce and the successful achievement of individual and organizational goals [6]. The recent pandemic underscored the value of a diverse and resilient healthcare workforce, particularly in the United States, where a heterogeneous group of healthcare providers proved to be more adaptable and effective in facing the crisis [7].

10.2 The Rational for Promoting Changes

The rationale for suggesting essential, recommended, and optional changes is funded on several facts:

(a) The ongoing gender gap in fellowships, authorships, grant success rates, and editorial positions in medical journals [8].
(b) Social bias exists not only in systems lacking awareness, but also in societies that are conscious of the issue [9]. For example, female scientists in Australia were less likely to win a major type of medical-research grants than their male counterparts, despite a gender equity push at the *National Health and Medical Research Council* [8]. The *Australian National Health and Medical Research Council* has acknowledged the problem in the past and in a gender strategy report released during the previous years the agency did allocate additional funding to a small number of female researchers [8].
(c) The gender gap in authorship and its implications for metrics like the H-index, which is widely used in perioperative and critical care medicine publications [10, 11].
(d) The absence of visible role models in medical literature and the lack of mentorship in the publication process are key issues. Editors of *Nature* and its associated journals have been working to strengthen existing initiatives on diversity, equity, and inclusion [12]. Gender disparities in publications have been shown to correlate with future academic rank signifying sustained impact on professional careers [13], salary and job satisfaction [14].

Reflection Point Recent studies have shown that pay transparency can significantly reduce inequities in the workplace [15]. How transparent is the pay structure in your hospital or institution? Are you aware of any efforts to address pay equity within your organization?

(e) The medical profession has seen a significant increase in the enrolment of women in medical schools [4]. Despite this objective data, it is unclear if most female graduates will perform any clinical work at the bedside. A scoping review has been started with the aim to investigate the extent of this disparity, understand its underlying causes, and propose potential engagement of this unvaluable resources in more flexible jobs such as "research coordinators" (unpublished data). Education, resources, and training of the workforce is difficult or inadequate without a knowledge of the composition and the need of the students.

(f) The need for a blame-free culture is represented in the ability to have incident reporting [16, 17]. A blame-free culture is one in which individuals feel able to report errors without fear of punishment. This permits more reporting of harmful incidents and near-misses, encourages more collaboration across disciplines, and allows a focus on finding systemic solutions [17]. At the core of the 2000 Institute of Medicine report *To Err is Human*, it is emphasized that "the problem is not bad people in healthcare—it is that good people are working in bad systems that need to be made safer." A blame-free culture is a key element of creating a "just culture." Fostering such a culture of tolerance is an essential step toward indirectly promoting DEI [18].

(g) There is a need for healthcare professionals to understand how self-critical beliefs can contribute to emotional distress in their patients [19]. By promoting DEI approaches in care, professionals can better understand the varied experiences of their patients, leading to more personalized support and interventions that address unique emotional and psychological needs. This inclusive perspective fosters empathy and helps create a supportive environment where all patients feel valued and understood, ultimately improving health outcomes [4].

10.3 The Changes

These changes are categorized into three tiers: essential, recommended, and optional (Table 10.1).

Essential changes include implementing policies that promote equitable hiring and retention practices. Abrogating the gender gap in all levels of academia are official priorities of the National Institutes of Health [20] and the European Commission [21].

It is essential to create international dataset to learn more about the nature (age, sex, gender, race, origin, religion, etc.) of the workforce standing at the bedside in perioperative and critical care medicine. Knowing the composition of bedside healthcare staff in high, upper-middle, lower-middle, and low-income countries could help guide education and provide targeted support for frontline workers in both their clinical practice and research.

Among the essential actions needed (Table 10.1), we can include promoting role models and adjusting performance metrics.

> **Reflection Point** Reflect on your educational experience—can you recall any female scientists in your science textbooks or female leaders in your history books? How might the representation (or lack thereof) of women in these contexts influence perceptions of gender roles in academia and leadership?

Table 10.1 Summary of actions needed

	Essential	Recommended	Optional
Recruitment	Job advertisements can be designed to be free from bias by using inclusive language that encourages diverse candidates to apply	Blind hiring practices that remove identifiable information (e.g., name, gender) from applications to reduce bias in hiring	Targeted recruitment of women in certain specialties and/or training programs
Promotions	Transparent criteria for promotions will ensure equitable opportunities for advancement	Mentorship and sponsorship opportunities for women employees, pairing them with senior staff who can guide and advocate for their career growth	Implementing mandatory gender ratios for promotions
Professional development	Equitable access to skill-building workshops, and continuing education. Modify H-index to adapt to new society needs and more inclusive workforce	Mandatory attendance at CME/CPD	Identifying skill gaps in women and offering targeted training workshops/ courses
Leadership training	Equitable access to leadership training workshops	Regularly train all employees on recognizing and addressing biases and understanding diverse cultural backgrounds	Targeted leadership courses for women
Organizational culture	Clear non-discrimination and anti-harassment policies	Anonymous channels for reporting discrimination or bias without fear of retaliation	Celebrate and acknowledge the contributions of employees from different backgrounds
Accountability	Regular reviews to identify and address pay disparities across gender, race, and other demographics	Set measurable goals for workforce diversity and regularly report progress to leadership and staff	Incorporate DEI-related goals into performance evaluations for leadership and staff
Overcome leaky pipeline (leadership development)	Collaborate with schools and community organizations to build interest in healthcare careers among underrepresented youth and women. Create new role models from primary education	Scholarships/grants for women and students from underrepresented backgrounds pursuing healthcare degrees	Paid internships and fellowships that prioritize women and candidates from diverse backgrounds

(continued)

Table 10.1 (continued)

	Essential	Recommended	Optional
Flexible and inclusive work policies	Flexible work schedules or telehealth opportunities to accommodate caregiving responsibilities of women in healthcare	Access to extended maternity and parental leave and support for mothers with young children	Daycare (nursery) facilities at hospital premises
Cultural barriers	Zero tolerance for harassment and abuse towards women HCW	Safe and secure accommodation for night duties	Pick and drop facilities in regions affected by conflict and wars is a critical measure to ensure the safety and mobility of women HCW

Abbreviations: *CME* Continuing Medical Education, *CPD* Continuing Professional Development, *HCW* healthcare workers

H-Index is a globally accepted metric which holds no correction factor to account for the possibility of having parental leaves [22]. Nevertheless, H-Indexes impact timing of promotion, but also tenure, salary, research funding, and appointment to leadership positions. This has been identified as one of the potential factors contributing to sex disparities in academic medicine [22]. Ha et al. [23] outline several systematic interventions that can positively impact the h-index disparity, specifically education, formal mentorship programs, career development programs, and institutional policies supporting work-life integration. In 2005, Jorge Hirsch proposed a new measure of research impact [24]. "A researcher's *h*-index is the number of his or her papers (*h*) that have been cited at least (*h*) times. In simple terms, a researcher with 10 published articles, each of which has received at least 10 citations, has a *h*-index of 10 [24]. "DORA", developed by the Centre for Science and Technology Studies (CWTS), examines bibliometric and scientometrics tools to support research assessment reform and inform strategic decision-making in the development of science policy. [25] By supporting research assessment reform and strategic decision-making in science policy, DORA encourages institutions, publishers, and funders to adopt more inclusive and transparent practices, ultimately promoting a fairer, more accurate system for assessing research and advancing science. This is crucial for fostering innovation, improving collaboration, and ensuring that diverse contributions, including those from underrepresented groups, are recognized and valued.

In addition, individuals and departments should sponsor women for scholarly opportunities, especially roles that lead to manuscript authorship, and their publications should be highlighted and promoted by their institutions [23]. Similar reflections could be done for race, ethnicity, LGBTQ+, and disabilities [23]. Set up policies and measurable actions are recommended to reach better equity, such as code of conduct policies similar to those adopted by the World Federation of Societies of Intensive and Critical Care Medicine [26, 27]. Widespread adoption of such policies would theoretically help eliminate inequity and enhance inclusion [28, 29].

Recommended changes involve providing training on unconscious bias including prevention of unconscious biases in various settings such as committees, job interviewing panels, editorial boards, grants evaluation committees, etc. It is our collective responsibility to identify and address barriers that perpetuate inequities in CCM [4]. To effectively address unconscious bias, it is crucial to first raise awareness, using tools like the Implicit Association Test to help individuals identify their biases [30]. Strategies to mitigate implicit bias include conducting simulations and debates that normalize discussions about bias as a common human tendency, and offering workshops that focus on recognizing unconscious bias through interactive clinical scenarios [31]. Anonymizing peer reviews in the editorial process can also be beneficial [4]. In this respect, it is important to note that women became members of the *Anesthesia & Analgesia* and *Anesthesiology* editorial boards in 1980 and 1987, respectively [31]. A recent paper reported an increased proportion of female ICU physicians in China [31] with a persistent wide gender gap. The authors pointed out that the biggest challenges faced by female ICU physicians include inadequate work-life balance, difficulties in career planning, and lack of academic support [32].

Optional initiatives may be mentorship/sponsorship programs or community outreach efforts to further support diverse talent development [33].

Optional Actions could be to implement facilities for childcare in the public service, mainly in the workplaces, such as maternity schools, bus/shuttle service, allowing parents to ensure the necessary care their children need while they are working, to allow parents to spend more time working in the academic or clinical field [33]. The implementation of facilities for childcare in the public service, mainly in the workplaces, would be a fundamental to support young couples at the start of their careers [4].

Furthermore, creating a safe learning environment—known as a "safe but brave" space—can establish ground rules that promote confidentiality and psychological safety, allowing participants to discuss challenging topics without fear.[34,] Finally, skill-building activities, such as role-plays, vignettes, and standardized patient interactions, can help individuals develop and practice the skills necessary to confront and address bias effectively [34].

There is also the need for healthcare professionals to understand how self-critical beliefs can contribute to emotional distress in their patients. Most studies indicate that self-blame is linked to increased emotional distress, particularly among individuals diagnosed with chronic physical health conditions such as cancer, HIV/AIDS, and cardiovascular disease [36, 37]. However, concerns about the quality of the reviewed studies may undermine the reliability of these findings [36]. Further research is necessary to understand the impact of self-blame on outcome. Self-blame relates to illness onset and its impact on distress and well-being.

Healthcare professionals must also recognize how self-critical beliefs can contribute to emotional distress in their patients [35]. Research indicates that self-blame is often linked to increased emotional distress, particularly in individuals with chronic conditions such as cancer, HIV/AIDS, and cardiovascular disease [36, 37]. However, the reliability of these findings may be questioned due to concerns about the quality of the studies reviewed [36]. Further research is needed to better understand how self-blame, particularly regarding illness onset, impacts patient outcomes, distress, and overall well-being.

In low-income countries (LIC) we can identify some specific actions to consider: essential, recommended, or optional. **The essential actions** are: clear non-discrimination and anti-harassment policies, regular reviews to identify and address pay disparities across gender, race, and other demographics, collaboration with schools and community organizations to build interest in healthcare careers among underrepresented youth and women, and zero tolerance for harassment and abuse towards women. **The recommended actions** include scholarships/grants for women and students from underrepresented backgrounds pursuing healthcare degrees, mentorship opportunities for women employees, pairing them with senior staff who can guide and advocate for their career growth, and blind hiring practices that remove identifiable information (e.g., name, gender) from applications to reduce bias in hiring. **The optional actions** to consider are: implementing mandatory gender ratios for promotions, identifying skill gaps in women and offering targeted training workshops/courses sponsored from high-income countries, celebrating and acknowledging the contributions of employees from different backgrounds, incorporating DEI-related goals into performance evaluations for leadership and staff, paid internships and fellowships that prioritize women and candidates from diverse backgrounds, pick and drop facilities in regions affected by conflict and wars is a critical measure to ensure the safety and mobility of women HCW.

Reflection Point Why do the essential, recommended, and optional actions for promoting DEI differ between low-income countries (LICs) and high-income countries (HICs)? What factors contribute to these variations in priorities, and how can LICs address these disparities given the unique challenges they face in terms of resources, infrastructure, and socio-political factors? How can we ensure that DEI initiatives are tailored to each country's context, while still aligning with global standards of equity and inclusion?

In conclusion, several strategies have been proposed to reduce the gap but still no decisive improvement has been detected. These solutions proposed at different levels should be implemented, tracked, and well-measured for the future and stratified for focused need in high, upper middle, lower middle, and low-income countries as identified by the World Bank [38].

Proposed Actions

1. **Implement Equitable Hiring Policies:** Establish and enforce policies that promote equitable hiring and retention practices across all levels of academia. This includes adopting blind hiring practices to minimize bias related to gender, race, and other demographics.
2. **Support Role Models and Mentorship:** Create formal mentorship programs and sponsorship initiatives that pair women and underrepresented individuals with senior staff. This will facilitate career development and increase visibility of diverse talent in leadership and authorship roles.
3. **Provide Training on Unconscious Bias:** Offer regular training sessions on unconscious bias for all staff involved in hiring, evaluations, and promotions. Utilize tools like the Implicit Association Test to enhance awareness and understanding of bias in various professional settings.
4. **Establish Safe Learning Environments:** Create "safe but brave" spaces within organizations where individuals can discuss challenging issues related to equity and diversity confidentially. Create a "just culture" and "blame-free incident reporting".
5. **Create datasets that identify bedside healthcare workers globally.** Knowing the workforce is easier to address the needs.

Follow the link to learn more about how **women are unused reservoir of recourses**. Reflect on implementation of change.

VIDEO LEGEND: "Francesca Rubulotta, in her presentation at the World Day of Critical Lung, explores the 'leaky pipeline' phenomenon in anesthesia and critical care, addressing whether women are an unused—or insufficiently utilized—reservoir of resources."

References

1. Gomez LE, Bernet P. Diversity improves performance and outcomes. J Natl Med Assoc. 2019;111:383–92.
2. Venkatesh B, Mehta S, Angus DC, Finfer S, Machado FR, Marshall J, Mitchell I, Peake S, Zimmerman JL. Women in intensive care study: a preliminary assessment of international data on female representation in the ICU physician workforce, leadership and academic positions. Crit Care. 2018;22(1):211. https://doi.org/10.1186/s13054-018-2139-1. PMID: 30196796; PMCID: PMC6130077.
3. Metaxa V. Is this (still) a man's world? Crit Care. 2013;17(1):112. https://doi.org/10.1186/cc11859. PMID: 23360566; PMCID: PMC3573347.

4. Vincent JL, Juffermans NP, Burns KEA, Ranieri VM, Pourzitaki C, Rubulotta F. Addressing gender imbalance in intensive care. Crit Care. 2021;25(1):147. https://doi.org/10.1186/s13054-021-03569-7. PMID: 33863353; PMCID: PMC8051087.
5. https://www.gmc-uk.org/-/media/documents/fair-to-refer-report_pdf-79011677.pdf
6. General Medical Council. Chapter3: the changing medical work force. 2020. Accessed 16 April 2021. https://www.gmc-uk.org/-/media/documents/somep-2020-chapter-3_pdf-84686032.pdf?la=en&hash=D2F3AD68AF8820D40A285BDC6A391A85A780C88B 2. Centre for Workforce Intelligence. Shape of the medical workforce: starting the debate on the future consultant workforce. February 2012. Accessed April 16 2021. https://assets.publishing.service.gov.uk/government/uploads/system/uploads/attachment_data/file/507651/CfWI_future_consultant_workforce.pdf.
7. Zhong L, Lopez D, Pei S, Gao J. Healthcare system resilience and adaptability to pandemic disruptions in the United States. Nat Med. 2024;30(8):2311–9. https://doi.org/10.1038/s41591-024-03103-6. Epub 2024 Jul 2. PMID: 38956198.
8. Nogrady B. Female researchers in Australia less likely to win major medical grants than males. Nature. 2019. Published on line October 22, 2019; https://doi.org/10.1038/d41586-019-03038-w.
9. Hart KL, Perlis RH. Trends in proportion of women as authors of medical journal articles, 2008–2018. JAMA Intern Med. 2019;179(9):1285–7. https://doi.org/10.1001/jamainternmed.2019.0907.
10. Vranas KC, Ouyang D, Lin AL, Slatore CG, Sullivan DR, Kerlin MP, Liu KD, Baron RM, Calfee CS, Ware LB, Halpern SD, Matthay MA, Herridge MS, Mehta S, Rogers AJ. Gender differences in authorship of critical care literature. Am J Respir Crit Care Med. 2020;201(7):840–7. https://doi.org/10.1164/rccm.201910-1957OC. PMID: 31968182; PMCID: PMC7124723.
11. Chary S, Amrein K, Soeteman DI, Mehta S, Christopher KB. Gender disparity in critical care publications: a novel female first author index. Ann Intensive Care. 2021;11(1):103. https://doi.org/10.1186/s13613-021-00889-3. PMID: 34213685; PMCID: PMC8253865.
12. Nature'sunder-representation of women. Nature 2018; 558 (7710):344. https://doi.org/10.1038/d41586-018-05465-7.
13. Carr PL, Raj A, Kaplan SE, Terrin N, Breeze JL, Freund KM. Gender differences in academic medicine: retention, rank, and leadership comparisons from the National Faculty Survey. Acad Med. 2018;93(11):1694–9. https://doi.org/10.1097/ACM.0000000000002146. PMID: 29384751; PMCID: PMC6066448.
14. Holden C. General contentment masks gender gap in first AAAS salary and job survey. Science. 2001;294(5541):396–411. https://doi.org/10.1126/science.294.5541.396. PMID: 11598304.
15. Obloj T, Zenger T. The influence of pay transparency on (gender) inequity, inequality and the performance basis of pay. Nat Hum Behav. 2022;6(5):646–55. https://doi.org/10.1038/s41562-022-01288-9. Epub 2022 Feb 10. PMID: 35145281.
16. Cooper J, Edwards A, Williams H, Sheikh A, Parry G, Hibbert P, Butlin A, Donaldson L, Carson-Stevens A. Nature of blame in patient safety incident reports: mixed methods analysis of a National Database. Ann Fam Med. 2017;15(5):455–61. https://doi.org/10.1370/afm.2123. PMID: 28893816; PMCID: PMC5593729.
17. Wu AW, Kachalia AB. Creating a "just culture": more work to be done. J Macromark. 2023;28(2):100–13. https://doi.org/10.1177/02761467211054836.
18. Institute of Medicine (US). Committee on quality of health Care in America. In: Kohn LT, Corrigan JM, Donaldson MS, editors. To err is human: building a safer health system. Washington, DC: National Academies Press (US); 2000.
19. Callebaut L, Molyneux P, Alexander T. The relationship between self-blame for the onset of a chronic physical health condition and emotional distress: a systematic literature review. Clin Psychol Psychother. 2017;24(4):965–86. https://doi.org/10.1002/cpp.2061. Epub 2016 Dec 7. PMID: 27925335.
20. National Institutes of Health (NIH) Gender Inequality Task Force. Addressing gender inequality in the NIH intramural research program action task force report and recommendations. National Institutes of Health (NIH) Gender Inequality Task Force; 2016.

21. European commission directorate-general for research and innovation. Gender equality: achievements in horizon 2020 and recommendations on the way forward. Publications Office, 2020. https://doi.org/10.2777/009204.
22. Larson AR. Implications of sex disparities in the h-index for academic medicine. JAMA Netw Open. 2021;4(6):e2112877. https://doi.org/10.1001/jamanetworkopen.2021.12877. PMID: 34185073.
23. Ha GL, Lehrer EJ, Wang M, Holliday E, Jagsi R, Zaorsky NG. Sex differences in academic productivity across academic ranks and specialties in academic medicine: a systematic review and meta-analysis. JAMA Netw Open. 2021;4(6):e2112404. https://doi.org/10.1001/jamanetworkopen.2021.12404.
24. Barnes C. The h-index debate: an introduction for librarians. J Acad Librariansh. 2017;43(6):487–94.
25. https://sfdora.org/resource/halt-the-h-index/ (consulted 9th December 2024).
26. European Institute for Gender Equality. Gender mainstreaming: a guide to organisational change. https://eige.europa.eu/gender-mainstreaming/toolkits/gender-institutional-transformation/gender-mainstreaming-guide-organisational-change. Accessed 3 March 2021.
27. Godier A, Nouette-Gaulain K, Cittanova ML, Beloeil H, Paugam-Burtz C, Lukaszewicz AC. Women in anaesthesia and intensive care medicine in France: are we making any progress? Anaesth Crit Care Pain Med. 2020;39:507–11. https://doi.org/10.1016/j.accpm.2020.04.019.
28. Burns KEA, Straus SE, Liu K, Rizvi L, Guyatt G. Gender differences in grant and personnel award funding rates at the Canadian Institutes of Health Research based on research content area: a retrospective analysis. PLoS Med. 2019;16:e1002935. https://doi.org/10.1371/journal.pmed.1002935.
29. Bismark M, Morris J, Thomas L, Loh E, Phelps G, Dickinson H. Reasons and remedies for under-representation of women in medical leadership roles: a qualitative study from Australia. BMJ Open. 2015;5:e009384. https://doi.org/10.1136/bmjopen-2015-009384.
30. Onyeador IN, Hudson STJ, Lewis NA. Moving beyond implicit bias training: policy insights for increasing organizational diversity. Policy Insights Behav Brain Sci. 2021;8(1):19–26. https://doi.org/10.1177/2372732220983840.
31. McMullen K, Kraus MB, Kosiorek H, Harbell MW. Representation of women as editors in anesthesiology journals. Anesth Analg. 2022;134(5):956–63. https://doi.org/10.1213/ANE.0000000000005881. PMID: 35073283.
32. Liao X, Yang Y, Francesca R, Kang Y, Rello J. Female representation in intensive care medicine: challenges and perspectives from China. J Intensive Med. 2022;2(2):89–91. https://doi.org/10.1016/j.jointm.2021.12.002. PMID: 36789189; PMCID: PMC9923977.
33. Rubulotta F. Advancing careers in critical care medicine: the power of sponsorship and mentorship. Lancet Respir Med. 2024;12(2):99–101. https://doi.org/10.1016/S2213-2600(23)00425-3. Epub 2024 Jan 5. PMID: 38190835.
34. Moussié R. Childcare services in cities: challenges and emerging solutions for women informal workers and their children. Environ Urban. 2021;33(1):117–30. https://doi.org/10.1177/0956247820987096.
35. Clapper TC, Leighton K. Incorporating the reflective pause in simulation: a practical guide. J Contin Educ Nurs. 2020;51(1):32–8. https://doi.org/10.3928/00220124-20191217-07. PMID: 31895468.
36. Fernandes M, Aurino E. Chapter 25: Identifying an essential package for school-age child health: economic analysis. In: Bundy DAP, Silva ND, Horton S, Jamison DT, Patton GC, editors. Child and adolescent health and development. 3rd ed. Washington (DC): The International Bank for Reconstruction and Development / The World Bank; 2017. PMID: 30212130.
37. Just Culture Decision Support Tool. VA National Center for Patient Safety. https://www.patientsafety.va.gov/docs/Just-Culture-Decision-Support-Tool-2022.pdf (2022, access 21 March 2023).
38. https://blogs.worldbank.org/en/opendata/world-bank-country-classifications-by-income-level-for-2024-2025

11 Academic Advancement in Critical Care Medicine: Arena for Practicing Gender Equity and Diversity

Charlotte Salmon Gandonnière, Jordi Rello, and Olfa Hamzaoui

Key Points from the Editors

- Women often face a disproportionate burden of domestic and family responsibilities, limiting their ability to focus on research and early career advancement. This leads to slower academic progression compared to their male colleagues, despite similar qualifications and potential.

Supplementary Information The online version contains supplementary material available at https://doi.org/10.1007/978-3-031-86286-1_11.

C. Salmon Gandonnière (✉)
Médecine Intensive Réanimation, CHRU de Tours, Tours, France

INSERM CIC 1415, CHRU de Tours, Tours, France

FEMMIR group for the SRLF Trial group, Tours, France

J. Rello
Universitat Internacional de Catalunya, Barcelona, Spain

CRIPS Research Group-Vall d'Hebrón Institute Research Ps Vall d'Hebron 119, AMI– 14a Planta, Barcelona, Spain
e-mail: jrello@crips.es

O. Hamzaoui
Service de Médecine Intensive-Réanimation Polyvalente, Hôpital Robert Debré, Centre hospitalo-universitaire de Reims, Reims, France

Unité HERVI Hémostase et Remodelage Vasculaire Post-Ischémie-EA 3801, Université de Reims, Reims, France
e-mail: ohamzaoui@chu-reims.fr

V. Neskovic, F. Rubulotta (eds.), *Diversity, Gender Equity and Inclusion in Critical Care and Perioperative Medicine*,
https://doi.org/10.1007/978-3-031-86286-1_11

- Critical care medicine, a relatively recent speciality, has historically been male-dominated. Despite a growing number of women entering the field, particularly among younger physicians, their representation in academic positions remains low.
- Most of the factors contributing to the gender gap are also involved in the lack of diversity and inclusion in academic medicine.

Main Objectives

After reading this chapter, you will be able to:

- Recognize the underrepresentation of women in academic critical care medicine and discuss how this is reflected in fewer publications, limited research funding, and reduced visibility in leadership and recognition.
- Understand why gender equity cannot be achieved automatically with an increase in the number of women in a medical speciality and recognize the need for strong institutional commitment and proactive, multifaceted policies to effectively address gender disparities.
- Evaluate the steps and strategies that have been shown to improve academic promotion opportunities for women and minorities.

Introduction

Critical care medicine is a relatively recent speciality and has been considered for a long time as a male speciality (historically male-dominated). In any medical speciality, faculty represent the visible part of the speciality, particularly for medical students; reaching an academic rank is also considered as the best career achievement. For those reasons, gender equity in academic medicine is a key subject.

11.1 Where Are Women in Academic Medicine?

In a survey conducted in 2017 among 27 CCM scholarly societies (mainly from high-income countries), the proportion of female intensivists was 37 ± 11% [1]. In the United States (US) in 2021, women represented 27.3% of the 14,142 intensivists, and 26.1% of the 42,220 anaesthesiologists [2]. However, this proportion tends to increase; for instance, in a recent demographic report published in 2021, in the French College of Critical Care (CeMIR college des enseignants en médecine intensive reanimation), women represented 31% of French intensivists, but almost half of them among the youngers were physicians (under 40 years old) [3]. In the same manner, the proportion of women rose from 26% to 37% among intensive care trainees between 2006 and 2017 in Australia and New Zealand [1].

Nevertheless, the proportion of female ICM professors remains dramatically low, whatever the country. In a recent publication by Le Boedec et al., analysing demographic data from the French authority in charge of physicians between 2015 and 2020, CCM ranked among the last quartile in terms of female professors. Indeed, women represented only 8.8% of CCM full professors (8/91) [4]. There was no perspective of short-term improvement, as the sex ratio was the same among associated professors (1 woman out of 12 associated professors, 8.3%). Comparatively, the global rate of female full professors was 22% (all specialities together) [4].

Actually, the feminization of medicine does not spontaneously promote women's access to academic careers. In the US, a recent publication using data from the Association of American Medical Colleges demonstrated that women-associated professors were less likely to be promoted to full professors than men, whatever the speciality (hazard ratio (HR) 0.77), and there was no improvement of the HR between 1979 and 2013 [5].

The problem of the glass ceiling for physician women, and the lack of access to academic career, is not specific to CCM and perioperative medicine as even more data exist for all medical specialities taken together. One can reasonably extrapolate those data to CCM, to explore the factors contributing to the gender gap in academic rank in ICM.

11.1.1 Publication Gap

Indeed, literature has largely described a persistent gender publication gap among academic physicians. All specialities confounded that in the US, the rate of female first authors among 6 prominent medical journals rose from 5.9% in 1970 to 29.3% in 2004; the rate of female last authors in the same journals rose from 3.7% to 19.3% [6].

Accordingly, Vranas et al. analysed 18,483 publications in the field of critical care, in the 40 frequently cited journals: the authors reported that 30.8% of the first authors were women, and only 19.5% were senior authors. Interestingly, a female senior author increased the chance of having a female as a first author (OR 1.93). In addition, women were more likely to publish in a lower-impact factor journal than men [7]. Similar results are reported by Chander et al., in a publication regarding 12 prominent journals from 2000 to 2022 (7 ICM journals and 5 general journals), with 24.6% of women as first authors, and 16.6% of senior authors [8].

The gender gap in Hirsh-index (h-index) is problematic, as this index is a classical mean of evaluation, and therefore taken into account for career advancement or hiring [9, 10]. Indeed, the h-index is a measure of impact using the number of publications and citations. It is calculated using the number of times one's publications are cited in the literature and the measure of their impact. An individual's number of citations and, therefore, h-index increases with the number of publications and time since publication.

Women anaesthesiologists had a lower h-index than men (4.72 vs 9.49 among professors), even after adjustment for faculty rank [9], but with the same number of citations per publication, suggesting an equal level of publications' quality [11]. Interestingly, along with the progression of the career, it has been reported that the publication gap decreases until, at last, an inversion. Accordingly, women produce a mean of 1.57 more annual publications than men in the latter stages of the career, among physicians of the Mayo Clinic [12–15]. For this reason, correcting the h-index by adjustment on career duration (m-quotient) may be more rewarding for women as the gender gap disappears [16, 17].

Reflection Point Can h-index create bias and discrimination? Who can benefit the most? Read the list of potential drawbacks of the h-index.

- Each citation of a multiauthor paper is credited to all authors.
- Multiple authors count the same citations inflating the overall citation count.
- Varying levels of contribution in multiauthor papers are not considered (unfair comparisons between authors of single- vs. multi-authored works).
- Adding authors with little to no contribution to enhance career prospects.

11.1.2 Gap in Grant Attribution and Financial Support

Women are less likely to apply for a highly retributing grant [18]. If they apply, women are less likely to be attributed a National Institute of Health (NIH) grant, and among recipients, they are less likely to receive a second NIH grant, leading to a restricted access to the highest levels of research funding (HR for being allocated the highest level of funding for women: 0.79) [19]. British data confirm this trend: in the United Kingdom (UK), 28% of infectious disease national grants are awarded to women, although there was a trend of progression between 1998 and 2009. The amount awarded was greater for men (179,389 £ versus 125,556 £) [20]. In another publication, Sege confirmed this gender gap for the amount of research grants [21].

Beyond research grants, female physicians, researchers, faculty and women with leadership position perceive significantly less salary, even after adjustment on speciality, academic rank and number of publications, as demonstrated by a survey performed among US recipients of a NIH grant; the salary gap reached—13,399 US $ [22, 23].

Dr. Claudia Goldin won the 2023 Nobel Prize in economy for her research on female employment and the gender pay gap. Goldin highlighted the **slow progress in closing the gender wage gap**, noting that while it once stemmed from **differences in education and occupation**, today it persists **even within the same jobs**, worsening for women **after the first child is born.** (Source: The Nobel Prize).

11.1.3 Lack of Mentorship

The lack of mentorship for women has been addressed by several authors [9, 14, 24]. At the same level of competence, young female researchers are less likely to be offered mentorship by their faculty [25], while mentorship is demonstrated to be a key contributor to career advancement [26]. Women need mentors, and moreover role models, that is to say mentors in whom they can identify themselves [27]. In a study among premedical students in the US, female students being attributed female surgical mentors were more likely to consider a surgical career [28]. The importance of women mentors for promoting women faculty is illustrated by Vranas in the aforementioned publication: women senior authors are more likely to publish with women first authors [7]. Beyond mentorship, being a white male from the upper socio-economic class is a clear advantage for career advancement, because knowing the social codes and networking are fundamental; for example, having a PhD parent induces a 25-fold increase in the chances of being a faculty [29]. This is illustrated by the concept of "hidden curriculum" [30, 31]. Beyond mentoring, social networking is a key component in medical career, and men are more inclined to networking than women [32].

11.1.4 Lack of Representation and Visibility

More generally, women suffer from a terrible lack of representation and visibility. As underlined by Mehta and colleagues, the sepsis-3 definition publication does not include a single woman! (and no member from low-income country either) [33, 34]. CCM international societies are mainly led by men; in a recent publication [1], Venkatesh et al. reported a very low proportion of women among the presidents of the main CCM societies between 2002 and 2017 (European Society of ICM (ESICM): 0/9, Australia and New Zealand Intensive Care Society 1/9, World Federation of Societies of Intensive and Critical care Medicine 1/5). The US Society of Critical Care Medicine performed better, with 7 SCCM presidents women among the 17 between 2000 and 2017 [1].

In 2016, women represented less than 30% of the editorial board members of all major CCM societies, except for the SCCM, thanks to an ambitious diversity policy [35, 36]. Furthermore, women are underrepresented in meeting programs, representing less than 50% of the speakers. In a recent publication, in 9 medical specialities in the US, including anaesthesia, women represented around 30% of the speakers; this percentage did not reflect the percentage of women in each speciality (sex ratio after normalization to workforce demographic ranging from 0.56 for medical students to 0.79 for faculty) [37]. In the field of neuroimmunology, it has been shown that meetings' organizers try to justify this gap with a theoretical lack of qualified female experts and opinion leaders [38]; Robyn Klein brilliantly demonstrated the contrary by dressing a list of female experts not invited, and by checking that their number and quality of scientific publications were at least as good as men's. Moreover, adopting a gender balance policy improves women's representation, as demonstrated by the comparison of two different scientific meetings, one with a gender policy, and one without [38].

In ICM, women representation in major scientific meetings remains low: the proportion of female faculty from 2015 to 2017 was between 15% and 16.9% for ESICM [1]. Nevertheless, the appointment of a task force and working group for diversity and equality of the ESICM in 2019 induced a progressive improvement in women representation [39]. In the US, the representation of female faculty in scientific meetings reached 29% and 27% in 2015 and 2017, respectively [1]. Interestingly, the proportion of female faculty in the College of Intensive Care Medicine of Australia and New Zealand meeting rose from 7.7 to 34% between 2015 and 2017 [1], the year of the publication of guidelines for achieving gender balance at CICM events [40].

In the scientific field, it has also been demonstrated that women are less likely to be proposed for a publication review [41]. The proportion of women in the editorial boards of the main medical journals remains dramatically low (11.5%), despite a trend for improvement in the last decades (1.4% in 1970 to 16% in 2005) [42]. In the main CCM journals, women represented 17.5% of the editorial boards in 2011 [43] and 23.6% in 2022 [44].

> By being underrepresented in key public domains such as meetings, guideline panels, and publications, women are not seen as opinion leaders, reinforcing the perception of critical care medicine (CCM) as a male-dominated specialty.

11.2 Why Such a GAP?

There are numerous factors contributing to women's lack of visibility (in terms of publication, funding, scientific meetings), and, at last, to the gender gap; those factors are represented in Fig. 11.1.

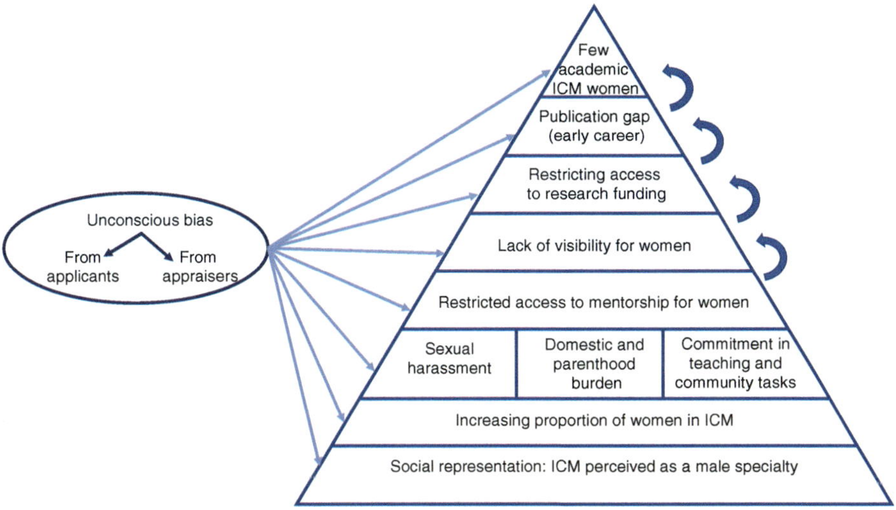

Fig. 11.1 Factors contributing to the gender gap in academic ICM. ICM: intensive care medicine

11.2.1 A Different Pathway

Several studies showed that women favour teaching occupation rather than research, while research is more rewarding for academic advancement [24, 45]. Moreover, women faculty dedicate more time than men to university services (tasks related to the good functioning of the institution), which could prevent them from advancing in their own research [46]. Likewise, in a publication concerning US anaesthesiologists, Pashkova et al. hypothesized that a greater contribution of women to clinical and educational tasks prevented them from being fully dedicated to their academic advancement [13].

11.2.2 Domestic and Family Charges

Additionally, the consistent finding that women's h-index overtakes men's h-index for later career steps tends to confirm a very unequal burden of domestic and family charges for young women. As academic advancement is determined early in young physicians, women clearly have unequal opportunities to achieve an academic career than their male counterparts [12, 14, 15].

In her study among US anaesthesiologists, Pashkova demonstrated that the burden of family care depended mainly on women [13]. Other studies in other specialities (otolaryngology, head and neck surgery, ophthalmology, radiation oncology, urology) retrieved similar factors contributing to the publication gap: family charge, greater interest in teaching. . . [14, 16, 47]. Indeed, it has been demonstrated that parenthood had a negative impact on women's career [48]. In a longitudinal survey among Swiss physicians from graduation to 7 years later, the authors reported that almost all part-time activities were occupied by women [48]. Both objective and subjective scales for career success achievement were worse for women than men, particularly for women with children. Indeed, there was no objective career penalization for men with children, while women with children experienced a worse career achievement. Both parenthood and the lack of mentor were associated with less satisfying career, and consequently women had to cross a double barrier as they had significantly less frequent mentors than men [48]. Seven years after graduation, female with children experienced a less advanced career than women without children or male. Parenthood was a factor preventing from choosing anaesthesia as a speciality, and females were less frequently candidates to an academic career than men [48].

Beyond the scope of medicine, demographic data evidence that women continue to dedicate more time to domestic and parenthood charges; a recent nationwide French survey reported 71% and 65% of domestic and parental burden undertaken by women, respectively [49]. Moreover, if women did reduce time allocated to domestic charges in the past 25 years, men did not increase their domestic charges, and both men and women increased their time dedicated to children care. As a consequence, the gender domestic gap barely reduced [49].

This has consequences on young researchers: among NIH grant recipients with active academic affiliation between 2006 and 2009, women dedicated 8.5 more hours per week to domestic activities than their male counterparts, after adjustment for work hours and partner employment. Similarly, women were almost 4 times more likely to adapt their schedule for childcare than men. Eighty-five percent of women had a full-time employed partner, versus only 45% of men [50]. In other words, academic women must endorse a double burden, domestic on the one side, academic on the other side.

Surveys among female intensivists (France, Australia, and New Zealand) report that despite a general satisfaction regarding quality of life, being a woman is perceived by one-third of the respondents as a disadvantage, particularly for academic advancement, and regarding pregnancy and breast-feeding issues [51, 52].

Reflection Point Men may wish different parental roles in today's societies. Can men who are more involved in family and childcare experience cultural bias and judgments? What is happening in your environment?

11.2.3 Unconscious Bias

It would be tempting to consider the gender gap in academic positions as a measurable phenomenon, attributable to a quantifiable insufficiency of women's achievements as compared to their male counterparts. Actually, an American publication demonstrated that women faculty have less publications, less first/last authorship, less NIH grants attributions, less trials registered in ClinicalTrails.gov than men; however, after multivariate adjustment on those parameters, women were still less likely than men to be promoted to full professors, in any speciality [53]. Other studies tend to confirm those data [54]. Among cardiologists, the OR of accessing a full professor rank after adjustment on those parameters was 0.63 [55]. Scientific data demonstrate that other complex factors are implied. Witteman et al. performed an interventional study among Canadian applicants for a federal grant between 2011 and 2016 (any field of research, clinical and fundamental, any speciality). There were two methods for project assessment and final decision of grant attribution: one method based in majority on the applicant's curriculum, and the second based in majority on the research project's quality. The gender gap for grant attribution was considerably reduced when the reviewers focused on the project rather than the applicant [56]. Thus, the quality of the research project is not responsible for the restricted access to grants for women. The remaining gap after adjustment on all measurable parameters is attributable to a sum of unconscious bias.

Unconscious bias is one of the main factors involved in the mechanisms leading to women discrimination and glass ceiling. An interesting experiment, performed in the field of mathematics, confirms this hypothesis. The authors evaluated the influence of gender on a hiring process [57]. Candidates of both sexes had to perform a mathematical test, known to be performed equally by men and women. When the only information available for employers was the physical appearance of the candidate, employers (whatever their sex) tended to hire a man rather than a woman. When the candidate self-reported the results to the test, men were still more frequently hired, because they tended to overestimate their performances while women tended to minimize their performances [57]. The gap was reduced by providing the full test results to employers. This demonstrates that implicit bias exists on both sides, from the candidates and from employers. The implicit association test (IAT) performed on employers confirmed the involvement of stereotypes in hiring discrimination. Women have to attest their competences even more because they start the hiring process with a clear disadvantage compared to their male counterparts [57]. Other publications in the scientific domains confirm the role of unconscious bias and support the imbalance of expectations towards women [25, 58–60] and African American researchers [58]. According to the implicit bias, women are considered more competent in social relationship (communal skills), while men are believed to be more efficient in task performance (agentic skills), a representation clearly advantaging in scientific disciplines [61]. A common stereotype is to consider that women do not have as many leadership skills as men [23]. Indeed, letters of recommendation for academic applicants tend to highlight communal qualities for women, and agentic qualities for men, reinforcing the stereotypes and the female disadvantage for faculty access [61].

The sum of all the bias and gender stereotypes in the field of science contribute to the well-known **"Matilda effect"** first described by Margaret Rossiter in 1993 [62]: in brief, women's research are frequently attributed to their male's counterparts, and women's contributions to scientific works are frequently omitted.

Because of this amount of bias, the efforts required for women are much higher to reach academic careers. Actually, the perception of gender bias and discrimination prevents women for considering an academic career [24].

Learn more about unconscious bias: Follow the link to a video with lecture explaining unconscious bias in more details.

VIDEO LEGEND: "Olfa Hamzai discusses implicit bias, its potential effects on clinical practice, and strategies for preventing it among healthcare professionals. Her presentation was part of the session at the World Day of Critical Lung, eighth edition, in 2024."

11.2.4 Aggression and Sexual Harassment

Women also have to deal with the risk of aggression and sexual harassment, at any timepoint of their career, from medical school and residency [24], to faculty [63, 64]. In a meta-analysis of 51 studies among medical trainees, 59% of the trainees reported at least one experience of harassment or discrimination, amongst which 33% of sexual harassment (the meta-analysis didn't provide sub-group analysis according to gender) [65]. In a survey among Australian and New Zealand fellows and trainees in ICM, 32% of the participants reported being bullied, 12% being discriminated, and 3% being sexually harassed. A small proportion (13%) of the cases of sexual harassment had been denounced. Women experienced a higher risk of being sexually harassed (OR 2.97) or discriminated (OR 2.1), but a similar risk to men of being bullied (OR 1.14) [66]. In academic ranges, this risk persists: in a survey among 1066 NIH awardees between 2006 and 2009, 30% of women and 4% of men reported sexual harassment [63]. Women faculty suffering from harassment may be assaulted by their mentors [67]. Previous data retrieved even more events, suggesting a trend in a reduction of sexual harassment prevalence, as 52% of female medical school faculty reported sexual harassment in 1995 [64]. In a 2022 report, the Association of American Medical Colleges (AAMC) stated an overall proportion of faculty experiencing sexual harassment of 22% (both women and men), and 34% among women [68]; the highest rates of sexual harassment among women faculty were in anaesthesiology and emergency medicine departments (52.6% each). Women suffering harassment were less satisfied and less committed in their institutions; they had a higher likelihood of leaving the institution [68]. Dealing with sexism and sexual harassment requires energy and affects productivity [69]; Zepeda called it "the harassment tax" [67, 70].

11.3 What About Diversity?

Most of the factors contributing to the gender gap are also involved in the lack of diversity and inclusion in academic medicine. From the beginning of medical school, racialized students suffer from microaggression and inner stereotypes [71]. Minorities are indeed underrepresented in academic ranks, as demonstrated by Riner et al. in the field of surgery; moreover, racialized women suffer from both gender and racial bias, and are the most penalized category [72]. There was no progression of Black and Hispanic proportion in academic ranks along the last 40 years [73]. Like for women, black-associated professors are less likely to be promoted to full professors compared to white counterparts (HR 0.74) [5]. Unfortunately, Richter's study did not analyse the potential additional effect of being a black woman. Like for woman, unconscious bias penalizes racial minorities: the expectations towards applicants differ according to their ethnicity [58].

Black researchers are 10% less likely than white researchers to be attributed a NIH grant, after adjustment on training, previous research awards, publications, and other demographic factors [74]. A multifaceted strategy for race bias awareness and correction has shown efficacy for bias reduction [75].

LGBTQ+ community also suffers inequity in the academic field. For example, sexual orientation represents a risk factor for experiencing sexual harassment, as both lesbian women and gay men had a 10% increase in the risk of being sexually harassed than their heterosexual counterparts [68].

Addressing a specific mentoring program for underrepresented minorities seems efficient for an improvement in diversity [26].

11.4 And Now, Time for Action!

We demonstrated above that women face more difficulties to achieve a good curriculum (publications, research grants). More perniciously, when they fulfil all the demands required for academic candidates, they still have a handicap compared to their men counterparts, because of unconscious bias and gender discrimination. As a consequence, it is unrealistic to expect gender equity to be "naturally" reached when the rate of women increases in a medical speciality [5]. Only a strong institutional commitment with proactive multifaceted policies can be efficient. Every

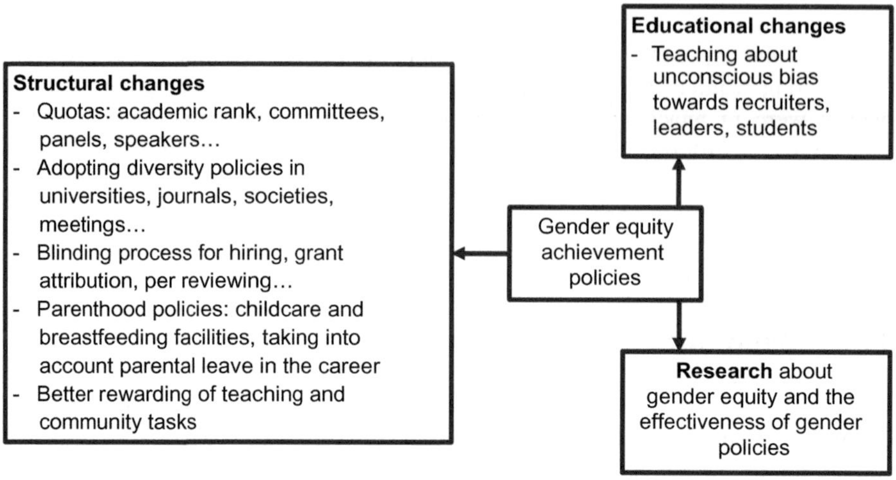

Fig. 11.2 Measures for gender equity achievement

arena for gender discrimination and bias listed above must be the field for ambitious measures for gender equality and diversity.

As Lucy Modra says, in ICU Management and Practice, "We cannot attract the highest quality leaders by recruiting from only half the pool of intensivists" [35]. Barriers to academic advancement for women deprive CCM from half of its potential leaders. We cannot afford such a waste!

The good news is that solutions exist, and many have been formalized by several institutions, mostly from Anglo-Saxon countries (US, UK, Australia, and New Zealand). Structural changes with multi-faceted policies must be preferred to individual enterprises for greater efficacy [35].

A multi-faceted intervention for women's promotion in academic medicine has demonstrated efficacy, as the percentage of women achieving the rank of associate professor rose with a proportion of 550% in 5 years, at John Hopkins University, in the 1990s [76].

Measures proposed for achieving gender equity are summarized in Fig. 11.2.

11.4.1 Academic Appointment and Hiring Policies

In the UK, the Athena swan charter for women's careers in higher education specifically promotes institutions committed in gender equity, particularly in the STEMM fields (sciences, technology, engineering, mathematics, and medicine). The Athena swan project attributes awards and provides institutional assistance to projects aiming at gender equity [77].

A study evaluated the existing programs for supporting, recruiting, promoting, and retaining women in academic medicine, in 24 American medical schools. Many institutions did not have a specific gender equity program. Existing programs focused mostly on individual and interpersonal levels. Childcare facilities and spousal hiring programs have been reported and seemed attractive for academic women. However, the authors insist on the lack of academic community measures, and the lack of specific policies [78].

Establishing quotas should be considered for enhancing diversity among faculty in CCM, at least during the period needed for achieving gender balance [35]. Data beyond the scope of medicine suggest that quotas induce gender heterogeneity resulting in an enhancement in the quality of work [79].

11.4.2 Filling the Publication Gap

Several measures have been proposed to reduce the publication gap. Among them, double-blinding the peer-review process could mitigate the effects of unconscious bias against female authors [35]. A recent systematic review of 8 publications retrieved an inconstant effect of this measure [80].

The editorial boards of the journals should achieve gender balance, and communicate about diversity metrics (rate of female board members, authors, first authors, senior authors), which should be easily available on their website [81]. For example, in Annals of Intensive Care, the review of the French Intensive Care Society (FICS) promotes women in its editorial board [82].

The way of reporting productivity should be challenged too; as described above, the h-index is disadvantaging for women, unlike the m-quotient which balances the number of publications with career duration [16]. This metric should be widely adopted.

11.4.3 Quality in Grant Awards/Fundings

Blinding grant attribution, parallel to the publications peer-review method, could be a way to overcome gender bias in research funding; Burke et al. retrieved an improvement, yet insignificant, in gender balance while anonymizing applications for a training program in Ireland [83].

11.4.4 Mentorship and Sponsorship

Having women as mentors and role models is fundamental [28]. Beech et al. published a review of published mentorship programs addressed for underrepresented minorities; although few objective outcomes are reported, such specific mentorship was satisfying for medical students, induced an increase in their productivity, and a greater academic career achievement [26]. Academic authorities should pay attention to mentor-mentee fit [84]. Mentorship network including women mentors, rather than a mentor-mentee duo, could also be a way to diversify role model [27].

If you are interested on more input about **Mentorship**, follow the link to watch the lecture on the same topic.

VIDEO LEGEND: "Florence Boissier, in her lecture at the eighth edition of the World Day of Critical Lung, explores the difference between sponsorship and mentorship in advancing women's careers."

11.4.5 Gender Equity in Scientific Meetings and Improving Women Visibility

The College of Intensive Care Medicine of Australia and New Zealand (CICM) published in 2017 guidelines for achieving gender balance at CICM events [40]. First, they recommend promoting women by fostering both merit AND gender, instead of choosing between merit and gender. Their aim was to reach 30% of female speakers for 2018's annual scientific meeting, 40% in 2020 and 50% in 2022, and diversity metrics must be published. The CICM specified that diversity must be attained for all sessions, and 100%-male panels have to be avoided as much as possible. The CICM encourages relationship with organizations aiming at achieving gender equity, such as the WIN network, Women in Intensive Care.

In the US, the NIH has published guidelines for funding scientific meetings if they are committed in gender equity and diversity such as the existence of a diversity plan that considers speakers, chairs, attendees, and organizing committee. The effectiveness of the plan must be reported. The guidelines also insist on the necessity of a safe and inclusive environment, with a specific focus on sexual harassment, and conference's accessibility for disabled attendees [85].

In general, women's visibility in academic medicine should improve in every field: speakers in meetings, editorial boards, but also in guidelines panels, committees, medical societies, exams evaluation panels, etc. [33]. Major ICM societies such as SCCM, ESICM, and national societies should display gender equity and communicate about that [81]. For instance, the French Intensive Care Society, the FICS, adopted a parity policy for its executive committee, effective since 2020, with an objective of full parity in 2023 [86]. Fifty per cent of CICM board members are women too [87]. As networking is a key factor for career advancement, women in ICM should gather in specific national and international network, such as the FEMMIR group of the French Intensive Care Society [81], or the international iWIN network, Women in Intensive Care.

11.4.6 Better Recognition of Less Rewarding Tasks

As it has been reported by several authors that academic women had greater involvement in teaching and in accomplishing university services [24, 45, 46], the institutions might set up measures in order to reward such involvement: for example, taking into account those kinds of commitments for academic promotion. In France, for example, the SIAPS score (score individuel d'aptitude à la pédagogie en santé, or individual score for health pedagogy skills) has been designed in order to evaluate applicants to an academic career on both research (publication index) and teaching skills [88].

11.4.7 Considering Family Charge

As domestic and family charge are still mostly assumed by women, raising children should be considered for career advancement. The expected h-index towards applicant could be adjusted regarding career breaks due to maternity leave and childcare. For instance, the allotted time for preparing an exam, a PhD, any academic file, should be prolonged after maternity leave (prolongation at least of duration as the maternity leave, but should probably be longer to balance the inequitable domestic charge).

> It is noteworthy that in order to reach gender equity, parental leaves should be encouraged (instead of maternity leave) and largely promoted all over the world, without conditions, for men and women [35].

Of course, it would be more desirable to reach complete gender equity in domestic and family burden, by promoting second parents' involvement in children and domestic care, but this major social shift will require decades, and as long as needed, measures must be taken to overcome this inequality.

As suggested by Carr, childcare facilities and partner hiring programmes may reinforce job attractivity for women [78]. Breast-feeding facilities could improve women's quality of life and promote pleasant motherhood at work [51].

As women won't stop having kids, there is an urgent need for a reduction in the unrealistic level of exigence towards academic candidates. Different profiles could be promoted for academic careers, some rather "scientific profiles", and other rather "teaching profiles", for example.

11.4.8 Circumvent Unconscious Bias

Actually, it has been shown that women apply for a job only if they fulfil 100% of the requirements, while men rather reach 60% of the requirements when they apply [89]. As a consequence, women tend to apply less frequently than men to job announcements [90]. Being aware of its own bias is the first step for reducing the impacts of this bias, particularly in the hiring process of scientists. Both applicants and recruiters must be trained to recognize bias: on the one side, women have to overcome bias preventing them from applying to a job [90]. On the other side, recruiters also have to struggle against their own bias as brilliantly demonstrated by Regner and colleagues [91]: denying having gender bias is worse than accepting them in terms of women's promotion. As an example, the Canadian Institute of Health Research provides a mandatory course about unconscious bias for peer reviewers [92]. It has been demonstrated in a cluster randomized controlled trial that providing faculty workshops about bias (gender-bias description, strategies to overcome bias) induced an increase in personal bias awareness, and an increase in the motivation for achieving gender equity [93].

In consequence, providing course about gender equity and implicit bias should be part of any medical curriculum, from premedical level to trainees, fellows, and faculty [33, 81]. Anyone could start by performing the Implicit Association Test (IAT), recognized as a reference for bias detection [94]. Workshops to improve women assertiveness should be also encouraged [81].

On a larger scale, the negative impact of the hidden curriculum has led the American College of Physicians to publish specific recommendations for shifting the hidden curriculum from negative to positive consequences: first, being aware of the cultural aspects of medicine is crucial, and ethical considerations, empathy, respect, inclusion, should be key principles in exercising medicine [31].

11.4.9 Ban Sexual Harassment

Sexual harassment must be banned, and a safe and diverse working atmosphere has to be promoted. Feeling secure at work fosters a better professional/personal balance and promotes women's productivity by refocusing their energy in their research work rather than avoiding behaviours. The AAMC published recommendations for addressing sexual harassment in academic medicine, both at the institutional and individual levels, in 2022 [68]. The American National Academy of Science, Engineering and Medicine (NASEM) published recommendations too, in 2018 [95]. Those 2 guidelines match for several crucial points: the need for a strong institutional commitment, the need for continuous training (for leaders, potential offenders, potential targets…), the need for transparency, the need of an adaptation of the hiring program, a clear and protocolized management of each situation (Table 11.1).

The main recommendations are summarized in Table 11.1.

Table 11.1 Main recommendations of the American Association of Medical Colleges and the National Academy of Science, Engineering and Medicine for addressing sexual harassment

	AAMC 2022	NASEM 2018
Hiring process	Actively seek for previous harassment reports regarding the applicant Hire faculty trained in management of sexual harassment	Promote gender and racial equity at every level
Institutional commitment	Have a multidisciplinary approach, involving faculty, human resources department, legal department, etc. Have local referents in each department. Imply department chairs Develop partnership with the parent university	Imply all levels of academy (e.g. medical societies) and the whole medical community.
Transparency policy	Centralize and communicate about sexual harassment reports	Communicate about institution's policy, transparency and accountability about each situation
Training	Training policy for faculty (management of situations) Educate both targets and offenders	Education, training (particularly towards leaders)
Management of reported situations	Address all inappropriate behaviour and inform about the sanctions incurred Adopt appropriate and proportionate sanctions	Adopt appropriate sanctions Measure the progress
Cultural aspects		Establish a cultural paradigm shift, beyond legal restrictions Support the targets of harassment
Research aspects		Attribute research grants in the field of gender diversity and sexual harassment

11.4.10 Promote Research in Gender Equity in CCM

As demonstrated above, providing literature about the gender gap allows to consider and measure the problem. However, few studies specifically evaluated the effect of gender gap correcting measures, although such studies are easy to design such as: before/after gender policy in one institution, randomized controlled trial in clusters comparing universities with or without gender policies, comparison of the sex ratio of journals according to the presence of a gender policy… Further research programs must be developed and funded, because filling the gender gap is not a question of conviction, but a matter of equity, justice, and a real scientific issue, necessary for a better care of patients and the improvement of work conditions for professionals [81].

11.5 Conclusion

Achieving gender equity and promoting global diversity and inclusivity benefits not only faculty and students but also enhances patient care. Therefore, it is crucial for all CCM institutions to implement comprehensive, multifaceted gender balance policies. Targeting these policies at the highest academic levels can be especially effective, as it creates a powerful role model effect that influences future generations of leaders in the field.

Proposed Actions

- Revise research productivity metrics, shifting from the h-index to more balanced measures like the m-quotient, which considers both publication output and career duration.
- Address gender bias in grant attribution by anonymizing applications and using blind assessments for research projects. Mandate unconscious bias training for peer reviewers.
- Increase women's visibility at scientific events by establishing guidelines. Report implementation and achieved diversity. Avoid all-male panels.
- Adjust career advancement metrics to account for parental leave and child-care responsibilities, ensuring researchers are not penalized for taking time off for family care.

References

1. Venkatesh B, Mehta S, Angus DC, Finfer S, Machado FR, Marshall J, et al. Women in Intensive Care study: a preliminary assessment of international data on female representation in the ICU physician workforce, leadership and academic positions. Crit Care. 2018;22(1):211.
2. AAMC. Active physicians by sex and specialty, 2021. Available from: https://www.aamc.org/data-reports/workforce/data/active-physicians-sex-specialty-2021
3. Ehrmann S, Guitton C, Aissaoui N, Terzi N, Capellier G, Vinsonneau C. Collège des Enseignants de Médecine Intensive Réanimation.
4. Le Boedec A, Anthony N, Vigneau C, Hue B, Laine F, Laviolle B, et al. Gender inequality among medical, pharmaceutical and dental practitioners in French hospitals: Where have we been and where are we now? PLoS One. 2021;16(7):e0254311.
5. Richter KP, Clark L, Wick JA, Cruvinel E, Durham D, Shaw P, et al. Women Physicians and Promotion in Academic Medicine. N Engl J Med. 2020;383(22):2148–57.
6. Jagsi R, Guancial EA, Worobey CC, Henault LE, Chang Y, Starr R, et al. The "gender gap" in authorship of academic medical literature--a 35-year perspective. N Engl J Med. 2006;355(3):281–7.
7. Vranas KC, Ouyang D, Lin AL, Slatore CG, Sullivan DR, Kerlin MP, et al. Gender differences in authorship of critical care literature. Am J Respir Crit Care Med. 2020;201(7):840–7.
8. Chander S, Luhana S, Sadarat F, Leys L, Parkash O, Kumari R. Gender and racial differences in first and senior authorship of high-impact critical care randomized controlled trial studies from 2000 to 2022. Ann Intensive Care. 2023;13(1):56.

9. Ha GL, Lehrer EJ, Wang M, Holliday E, Jagsi R, Zaorsky NG. Sex differences in academic productivity across academic ranks and specialties in academic medicine: a systematic review and meta-analysis. JAMA Netw Open. 2021;4(6):e2112404.
10. Braithwaite J, Herkes J, Churruca K, Long JC, Pomare C, Boyling C, et al. Comprehensive researcher achievement model (CRAM): a framework for measuring researcher achievement, impact and influence derived from a systematic literature review of metrics and models. BMJ Open. 2019;9(3):e025320.
11. Pagel PS, Hudetz JA. An analysis of scholarly productivity in United States academic anaesthesiologists by citation bibliometrics. Anaesthesia. 2011;66(10):873–8.
12. Reed DA, Enders F, Lindor R, McClees M, Lindor KD. Gender differences in academic productivity and leadership appointments of physicians throughout academic careers. Acad Med. 2011;86(1):43–7.
13. Pashkova AA, Svider PF, Chang CY, Diaz L, Eloy JA, Eloy JD. Gender disparity among US anaesthesiologists: are women underrepresented in academic ranks and scholarly productivity? Acta Anaesthesiol Scand. 2013;57(8):1058–64.
14. Eloy JA, Svider P, Chandrasekhar SS, Husain Q, Mauro KM, Setzen M, et al. Gender disparities in scholarly productivity within academic otolaryngology departments. Otolaryngol–Head Neck Surg. 2013;148(2):215–22.
15. Lopez SA, Svider PF, Misra P, Bhagat N, Langer PD, Eloy JA. Gender differences in promotion and scholarly impact: an analysis of 1460 academic ophthalmologists. J Surg Educ. 2014;71(6):851–9.
16. Mayer EN, Lenherr SM, Hanson HA, Jessop TC, Lowrance WT. Gender differences in publication productivity among academic urologists in the United States. Urology. 2017;103:39–46.
17. Khan NR, Thompson CJ, Taylor DR, Venable GT, Wham RM, Michael LM, et al. An analysis of publication productivity for 1225 academic neurosurgeons and 99 departments in the United States. J Neurosurg. 2014;120(3):746–55.
18. Waisbren SE, Bowles H, Hasan T, Zou KH, Emans SJ, Goldberg C, et al. Gender differences in research grant applications and funding outcomes for medical school faculty. J Women's Health. 2008;17(2):207–14.
19. Jagsi R, Motomura AR, Griffith KA, Rangarajan S, Ubel PA. Sex differences in attainment of independent funding by career development awardees. Ann Intern Med. 2009;151(11):804–11.
20. Head MG, Fitchett JR, Cooke MK, Wurie FB, Atun R. Differences in research funding for women scientists: a systematic comparison of UK investments in global infectious disease research during 1997–2010. BMJ Open. 2013;3(12):e003362.
21. Sege R, Nykiel-Bub L, Selk S. Sex Differences in Institutional Support for Junior Biomedical Researchers. JAMA. 2015;314(11):1175–7.
22. Jagsi R, Griffith KA, Stewart A, Sambuco D, DeCastro R, Ubel PA. Gender differences in the salaries of physician researchers. JAMA. 2012;307(22):2410–7.
23. Hastie MJ, Lee A, Siddiqui S, Oakes D, Wong CA. Misconceptions about women in leadership in academic medicine. Can J Anaesth. 2023;17:1–7.
24. Edmunds LD, Ovseiko PV, Shepperd S, Greenhalgh T, Frith P, Roberts NW, et al. Why do women choose or reject careers in academic medicine? A narrative review of empirical evidence. Lancet. 2016;388(10062):2948–58.
25. Moss-Racusin CA, Dovidio JF, Brescoll VL, Graham MJ, Handelsman J. Science faculty's subtle gender biases favor male students. Proc Natl Acad Sci USA. 2012;109(41):16474–9.
26. Beech BM, Calles-Escandon J, Hairston KG, Langdon SE, Latham-Sadler BA, Bell RA. Mentoring programs for underrepresented minority faculty in academic medical centers: a systematic review of the literature. Acad Med. 2013;88(4):541–9.
27. DeCastro R, Sambuco D, Ubel PA, Stewart A, Jagsi R. Mentor networks in academic medicine: moving beyond a dyadic conception of mentoring for junior faculty researchers. Acad Med. 2013;88(4):488–96.
28. Naimi BR, Bajaj V, Wang J, Litle VR, Merrill AL. The role of gender-concordant mentorship in women premedical students' perception and pursuit of surgical careers. J Surg Educ. 2023;S1931–7204(23):00177-0.

29. Morgan AC, LaBerge N, Larremore DB, Galesic M, Brand JE, Clauset A. Socioeconomic roots of academic faculty. Nat Hum Behav. 2022;6(12):1625–33.
30. Torres Acosta MA, Chandra S, Li S, Yoon E, Selgrade D, Quinn J, et al. The impact of underrepresented minority or marginalized identity status on training outcomes of MD-PhD students. BMC Med Educ. 2023;23(1):428.
31. Lehmann LS, Sulmasy LS, Desai S. Hidden curricula, ethics, and professionalism: optimizing clinical learning environments in becoming and being a physician: a position paper of the American college of physicians. Ann Intern Med. 2018;168(7):506–8.
32. Massen JJM, Bauer L, Spurny B, Bugnyar T, Kret ME. Sharing of science is most likely among male scientists. Sci Rep. 2017;7(1):12927.
33. Mehta S, Burns KEA, Machado FR, Fox-Robichaud AE, Cook DJ, Calfee CS, et al. Gender parity in critical care medicine. Am J Respir Crit Care Med. 2017;196(4):425–9.
34. Singer M, Deutschman CS, Seymour CW, Shankar-Hari M, Annane D, Bauer M, et al. The third international consensus definitions for sepsis and septic shock (Sepsis-3). JAMA. 2016;315(8):801–10.
35. Modra LJ, Yong SA. Women in leadership in intensive care medicine. ICU Manag Prac. 2016;16(3) HealthManagement.org. Radiology Management, ICU Management, Healthcare IT, Cardiology Management, Executive Management. Available from: https://healthmanagement.org/c/icu/issuearticle/women-in-leadership-in-intensive-care-medicine
36. Society of Critical Care Medicine (SCCM) | About SCCM. Available from: https://sccm.org/About-SCCM
37. Boiko JR, Anderson AJM, Gordon RA. Representation of Women Among Academic Grand Rounds Speakers. JAMA Intern Med. 2017;177(5):722–4.
38. Klein RS, Voskuhl R, Segal BM, Dittel BN, Lane TE, Bethea JR, et al. Speaking out about gender imbalance in invited speakers improves diversity. Nat Immunol. 2017;18(5):475–8.
39. Weiss B. Task force and working groups for diversity and equality of the ESICM. Statement paper on diversity for the European Society of Intensive Care Medicine (ESICM). Intensive Care Med. 2019;45(7):1002–5.
40. IC-28-Guidelines-for-Achieving-Gender-Balance-at-CICM-Events.pdf. Available from: https://www.cicm.org.au/CICM_Media/CICMSite/CICM-Website/Resources/Professional%20Documents/IC-28-Guidelines-for-Achieving-Gender-Balance-at-CICM-Events.pdf
41. Lerback J, Hanson B. Journals invite too few women to referee. Nature. 2017;541(7638):455–7.
42. Jagsi R, Tarbell NJ, Henault LE, Chang Y, Hylek EM. The Representation of Women on the Editorial Boards of Major Medical Journals: A 35-Year Perspective. Arch Intern Med. 2008;168(5):544–8.
43. Amrein K, Langmann A, Fahrleitner-Pammer A, Pieber TR, Zollner-Schwetz I. Women underrepresented on editorial boards of 60 major medical journals. Gend Med. 2011;8(6):378–87.
44. Yakar MN, Köşker RK, İbişoğlu E, Kara F, Hancı V. Gender distribution of editorial board members in critical care journals: assessment of gender parity. J Crit Care. 2023;75:154288.
45. Andriole DA, Jeffe DB. The road to an academic medicine career: a national cohort study of male and female U.S. medical graduates. Acad Med. 2012;87(12):1722–33.
46. Guarino CM, Borden VMH. Faculty service loads and gender: are women taking care of the academic family? Res High Educ. 2017;58(6):672–94.
47. Choi M, Fuller CD, Thomas CR. Estimation of citation-based scholarly activity among radiation oncology faculty at domestic residency-training institutions: 1996–2007. Int J Radiat Oncol Biol Phys. 2009;74(1):172–8.
48. Buddeberg-Fischer B, Stamm M, Buddeberg C, Bauer G, Hämmig O, Knecht M, et al. The impact of gender and parenthood on physicians' careers – professional and personal situation seven years after graduation. BMC Health Serv Res. 2010 Feb;18(10):40.
49. Champagne C, Pailhé A, Solaz A. Le temps domestique et parental des hommes et des femmes: quels facteurs d'évolutions en 25 ans ? Économie et Statistique 478-479-480 2015 | Insee. Available from: https://www.insee.fr/fr/statistiques/1303232?sommaire=1303240

50. Jolly S, Griffith KA, DeCastro R, Stewart A, Ubel P, Jagsi R. Gender differences in time spent on parenting and domestic responsibilities by high-achieving young physician-researchers. Ann Intern Med. 2014;160(5):344–53.
51. Hauw-Berlemont C, Aubron C, Aissaoui N, Bodet-Contentin L, Boissier F, Fartoukh MS, et al. Perceived inequity, professional and personal fulfillment by women intensivists in France. Ann Intensive Care. 2021;11(1):72.
52. Hawker FH. Female specialists in intensive care medicine: job satisfaction, challenges and work-life balance. Crit Care Resusc 2016 J;18(2):125–131.
53. Jena AB, Khullar D, Ho O, Olenski AR, Blumenthal DM. Sex differences in academic rank in US medical schools in 2014. JAMA. 2015;314(11):1149–58.
54. Carr PL, Raj A, Kaplan SE, Terrin N, Breeze JL, Freund KM. Gender differences in academic medicine: retention, rank, and leadership comparisons from the national faculty survey. Acad Med. 2018;93(11):1694–9.
55. Blumenthal DM, Olenski AR, Yeh RW, DeFaria YD, Sarma A, Stefanescu Schmidt AC, et al. Sex differences in faculty rank among academic cardiologists in the United States. Circulation. 2017;135(6):506–17.
56. Witteman HO, Hendricks M, Straus S, Tannenbaum C. Are gender gaps due to evaluations of the applicant or the science? A natural experiment at a national funding agency. Lancet. 2019;393(10171):531–40.
57. Reuben E, Sapienza P, Zingales L. How stereotypes impair women's careers in science. Proc Natl Acad Sci USA. 2014;111(12):4403–8.
58. Leslie SJ, Cimpian A, Meyer M, Freeland E. Expectations of brilliance underlie gender distributions across academic disciplines. Science. 2015;347(6219):262–5.
59. Smyth FL, Nosek BA. On the gender-science stereotypes held by scientists: explicit accord with gender-ratios, implicit accord with scientific identity. Front Psychol. 2015;6:415.
60. Isaac C, Lee B, Carnes M. Interventions that affect gender bias in hiring: a systematic review. Acad Med. 2009;84(10):1440–6.
61. Madera JM, Hebl MR, Martin RC. Gender and letters of recommendation for academia: agentic and communal differences. J Appl Psychol. 2009;94(6):1591–9.
62. Rossiter MW. The Matthew Matilda Effect in Science. Soc Stud Sci. 1993;23(2):325–41.
63. Jagsi R, Griffith KA, Jones R, Perumalswami CR, Ubel P, Stewart A. Sexual Harassment and Discrimination Experiences of Academic Medical Faculty. JAMA. 2016;315(19):2120–1.
64. Carr PL, Ash AS, Friedman RH, Szalacha L, Barnett RC, Palepu A, et al. Faculty perceptions of gender discrimination and sexual harassment in academic medicine. Ann Intern Med. 2000;132(11):889–96.
65. Fnais N, Soobiah C, Chen MH, Lillie E, Perrier L, Tashkhandi M, et al. Harassment and discrimination in medical training: a systematic review and meta-analysis. Acad Med. 2014;89(5):817–27.
66. Venkatesh B, Corke C, Raper R, Pinder M, Stephens D, Joynt G, et al. Prevalence of bullying, discrimination and sexual harassment among trainees and Fellows of the College of Intensive Care Medicine of Australia and New Zealand. Crit Care Resusc. 2016;18(4):230–4.
67. Murphy M, Record H, Callander JK, Dohan D, Grandis JR. Mentoring relationships and gender inequities in academic medicine: findings from a multi-institutional qualitative study. Acad Med. 2022;97(1):136–42.
68. AAMC. Understanding and addressing sexual harassment in academic medicine. Available from: https://www.aamc.org/data-reports/faculty-institutions/report/understanding-and-addressing-sexual-harassment-academic-medicine
69. Lindquist C, McKay T. Sexual harassment experiences and consequences for women faculty in science, engineering, and medicine. In: RTI press policy brief. Research Triangle Park (NC): RTI Press; 2010. Available from: http://www.ncbi.nlm.nih.gov/books/NBK542738/.
70. Zepeda L. The harassment tax. Science. 2018;359(6371):126.
71. Bullock JL, Lockspeiser T, Del Pino-Jones A, Richards R, Teherani A, Hauer KE. They don't see a lot of people my color: a mixed methods study of racial/ethnic stereotype threat among medical students on core clerkships. Acad Med. 2020;95(11S Association of American

Medical Colleges Learn Serve Lead: Proceedings of the 59th Annual Research in Medical Education Presentations):S58–66.
72. Riner AN, Herremans KM, Neal DW, Johnson-Mann C, Hughes SJ, McGuire KP, et al. Diversification of Academic Surgery, Its Leadership, and the Importance of Intersectionality. JAMA Surg. 2021;156(8):748–56.
73. Odei BC, Jagsi R, Diaz DA, Addison D, Arnett A, Odei JB, et al. Evaluation of equitable racial and ethnic representation among departmental chairs in academic medicine, 1980–2019. JAMA Netw Open. 2021;4(5):e2110726.
74. Ginther DK, Schaffer WT, Schnell J, Masimore B, Liu F, Haak LL, et al. Race, ethnicity, and NIH research awards. Science. 2011;333(6045):1015–9.
75. Devine PG, Forscher PS, Austin AJ, Cox WTL. Long-term reduction in implicit race bias: A prejudice habit-breaking intervention. J Exp Soc Psychol. 2012;48(6):1267–78.
76. Fried LP, Francomano CA, MacDonald SM, Wagner EM, Stokes EJ, Carbone KM, et al. Career development for women in academic medicine: Multiple interventions in a department of medicine. JAMA. 1996;276(11):898–905.
77. Athena Swan Charter | Advance HE. Available from: https://www.advance-he.ac.uk/equality-charters/athena-swan-charter
78. Carr PL, Gunn C, Raj A, Kaplan S, Freund KM. Recruitment, promotion, and retention of women in academic medicine: how institutions are addressing gender disparities. Womens Health Issues. 2017;27(3):374–81.
79. Dhir AA. Challenging boardroom homogeneity: corporate law, governance, and diversity. Cambridge: Cambridge University Press; 2015. Available from: https://www.cambridge.org/core/books/challenging-boardroom-homogeneity/A26334F8F5B99AF2A40DF5C869906D69
80. Kern-Goldberger AR, James R, Berghella V, Miller ES. The impact of double-blind peer review on gender bias in scientific publishing: a systematic review. Am J Obstet Gynecol. 2022;227(1):43–50.e4.
81. Hamzaoui O, Boissier F, Salmon Gandonnière C, Aubron C, Bodet-Contentin L, Fartoukh MS, et al. Ten actions to achieve gender equity among intensivists: the French Society of Intensive Care (FICS) model. Ann Intensive Care. 2022;12(1):59.
82. SpringerOpen. Annals of intensive care. Available from: https://annalsofintensivecare.springeropen.com/aoic-sdg5
83. Burke E, Heron EA, Hennessy M. Gender bias in academic medicine: a resumé study. BMC Med Educ. 2023;23(1):291.
84. Carapinha R, Ortiz-Walters R, McCracken CM, Hill EV, Reede JY. Variability in women faculty's preferences regarding mentor similarity: a multi-institution study in academic medicine. Acad Med. 2016;91(8):1108–18.
85. NOT-OD-21-053: Updated guidelines for enhancing diversity and creating safe environments in conferences supported by NIH grants and cooperative agreements. Available from: https://grants.nih.gov/grants/guide/notice-files/NOT-OD-21-053.html
86. SRLF. CA et Commissions. Available from: https://www.srlf.org/srlf/ca-commissions
87. CICM – Gender Equity – International Women's Day report 2023 from WIN. Available from: https://www.cicm.org.au/News-Summary/Gender-Equity-%E2%80%93-International-Women%E2%80%99s-Day-report-2
88. Roché H. Évaluer les compétences en pédagogie des candidats à des postes d'enseignants en médecine. Oncologie. 2016;18(6):361–2.
89. Mohr TS. Why women don't apply for jobs unless they're 100% qualified. Harv Bus Rev. 2014; Available from: https://hbr.org/2014/08/why-women-dont-apply-for-jobs-unless-theyre-100-qualified
90. Gender-Insights-Report.pdf. Available from: https://business.linkedin.com/content/dam/me/business/en-us/talent-solutions-lodestone/body/pdf/Gender-Insights-Report.pdf
91. Régner I, Thinus-Blanc C, Netter A, Schmader T, Huguet P. Committees with implicit biases promote fewer women when they do not believe gender bias exists. Nat Hum Behav. 2019;3(11):1171–9.

92. Government of Canada CI of HR. IGH Learning - CIHR. 2015. Available from: https://cihr-irsc.gc.ca/e/49347.html
93. Carnes M, Devine PG, Baier Manwell L, Byars-Winston A, Fine E, Ford CE, et al. The effect of an intervention to break the gender bias habit for faculty at one institution: a cluster randomized, controlled trial. Acad Med. 2015;90(2):221–30.
94. Project implicit. Available from: https://implicit.harvard.edu/implicit/
95. Johnson PA, Widnall SE, Benya FF, editors. Sexual harassment of women: climate, culture, and consequences in academic sciences, engineering, and medicine. Washington, D.C.: National Academies Press; 2018. Available from: https://www.nap.edu/catalog/24994

Implementation of Gender Equity and Diversity in Curricula of Critical Care and Perioperative Medicine

12

Beatrice Beck-Schimmer, Martin Schläpfer, Ulrike Weber-Stadlbauer, and Suzana Atanasoski

Key Points from the Editors

- **Revising medical school curricula and residency programs**: Medical education should begin by recognizing key differences between men and women in areas such as genetics, hormones, cardiovascular and respiratory function, immune response, inflammation, renal function, fertility, and psychological reactions to surgery. Then, it should be evaluated how these differences are currently addressed in existing programs.
- **Training in communication and inclusive language**: Medical professionals must be trained in communication skills and inclusive language to prevent stigmatization and discrimination in their daily interactions with patients and their families and colleagues.
- **Continuous education and feedback**: In addition to revising curricula, ongoing education and feedback are essential for lifelong learning, helping healthcare professionals develop competencies that promote an inclusive and fair working environment.

B. Beck-Schimmer (✉)
Institute of Anaesthesiology, University Hospital Zurich, University of Zurich, Zurich, Switzerland
e-mail: beatrice.beckschimmer@uzh.ch

M. Schläpfer
Institute of Anaesthesiology, University Hospital Zurich, Institute of Physiology, University of Zurich, Zurich, Switzerland
e-mail: martin.schlaepfer@uzh.ch

U. Weber-Stadlbauer · S. Atanasoski
University Medicine Zurich, University of Zurich, Zurich, Switzerland
e-mail: ulrike.weber@uzh.ch; suzana.atanasoski@uzh.ch

V. Neskovic, F. Rubulotta (eds.), *Diversity, Gender Equity and Inclusion in Critical Care and Perioperative Medicine*,
https://doi.org/10.1007/978-3-031-86286-1_12

Main Objectives
After reading this chapter, you will be able to:

- Explain the importance of integrating sex-specific differences into both preclinical and clinical medical curricula to enhance understanding and treatment of men and women.
- List key ethical and sociocultural competencies needed in clinical practice, including informed consent, decision-making, care for vulnerable patient groups, addressing religious beliefs, and end-of-life decisions.
- Recognize principles of faculty development and continuous medical education in promoting diversity, equity, and inclusion within healthcare settings.

12.1 Introduction

Implementing gender equity and diversity in the curricula of critical care and perioperative medicine requires a comprehensive, multifaceted approach. This involves not only addressing the physiological differences between sexes but also examining the broader societal, cultural, and leadership factors that contribute to gender-based disparities in healthcare. A key starting point is to review current curricula to identify gaps in equity and diversity-related topics, followed by the integration of gender-inclusive principles throughout all relevant courses and training modules.

In this chapter, we explore the gender differences that affect critical care and perioperative medicine and offer recommendations for education and research aimed at advancing gender equity and diversity in these fields.

12.2 Sex-Specific Anatomy and Physiology

While women and men undoubtedly share numerous anatomical and physiological similarities, behind this apparent symmetry lie important differences that significantly impact clinical approaches, treatment strategies, and outcomes. The differences stem from a combination of genetic variations, sex hormones, and the interplay of genetics and hormones themselves, which ultimately result in distinct physiological characteristics.

The human body composition varies across sexes [1]. Men typically exhibit a greater abundance of muscle and bone mass, while women tend to possess a higher percentage of body fat. Hormones play an important role in this disparity by causing several structural and morphological dissimilarities between the sexes, which in turn impact physiological functions. Another layer of complexity emerges from the shifting role of hormones across development as highlighted by Blair [1].

In the context of ***critical care and perioperative medicine,*** it is essential to address the following key factors: ***Firstly,*** it is important to recognize that female hearts typically have a smaller left ventricular mass and chamber size than men [1]. Their blood pressure varies over time with a rise in the postmenopausal phase. In addition, blood pressure regulation differs with women presenting reduced tolerance to impaired venous return. These variances have a notable impact on hemodynamic, fluid resuscitation, and drug dosing. Moreover, hormonal fluctuations exert a significant influence on heart rate [2], blood pressure, and clotting mechanisms [3], underscoring the need for gender-specific monitoring and interventions.

Secondly, sex-based disparities in lung size and capacity have direct implications for ventilator management and oxygenation strategies, while hormonal variations can also affect respiratory drive and response to mechanical ventilation [4].

Thirdly, estrogen and progesterone play an important role in immune response and inflammation, but also in infection susceptibility [5]. Also, one must consider the hormonal fluctuations during the menstruation cycle, pregnancy, and menopause when defining strategies for female patients.

Finally, sex-related variations in renal function including drug clearance impact on the dosing of medication and the application of fluids [6].

In ***perioperative medicine*** disparities across genders bear significant implications for surgical planning, but also for potential complications [1–6]. Hormones further impact on wound healing, coagulation, and immune response post-surgery. The use of hormonal contraception and hormone replacement therapy indirectly affects anesthesia and, most importantly, clotting factors. Moreover, hormonal and genetic factors contribute to different pain profiles in females, demanding careful consideration in pain assessment and management protocols. Pregnancy status is essential to anesthesia, monitoring, and appropriate patient positioning during surgery. Concerns related to fertility and patient preferences regarding reproductive organs should be part of the equation.

Beyond the physical aspects, gender roles, body image, and psychological responses to surgery can profoundly impact the patient's journey during the medical treatment and recovery phase.

Reflection Point Despite the importance of sex-based differences in physiology, these are typically not systematically addressed in physiology textbooks or medical curricula, except for reproductive physiology. What is your impression of this gap? Was this topic ever discussed during your training?

12.3 Sex-Specific Pharmacology

The primary objective when prescribing a specific medication should be to optimize therapeutic outcomes while mitigating negative effects. The interplay of pharmacokinetics and pharmacodynamics is pivotal in achieving this objective, and it is worth noting that these factors might be different between sexes [7–9]. Variations exist between men and women in the way drugs are absorbed through body surfaces such as the respiratory, gastrointestinal, or dermal tract. This is attributed to differences in pulmonary function, gastric emptying, and dermal thickness, among other factors. Moreover, anatomical distinctions between females and males, encompassing body weight, height, total body water, as well as extracellular and intracellular water, impact the distribution of drugs throughout the body [10]. Metabolism, primarily occurring in the liver through enzymes like the CYP group, exhibits significant differences between men and women [11]. Similarly, renal drug clearance, involving variations in glomerular filtration, tubular secretion, and tubular reabsorption, differs between sexes [9]. Both metabolism and renal clearance contribute to a drug's half-life and consequently influence potential adverse events.

Similar gender-based differences extend to pharmacodynamics as well. The responsiveness of receptors to medications can diverge between males and females due to hormonal influences, affecting drug-receptor binding and subsequent cellular responses [7–9].

> Considering differences in pharmacokinetics and pharmacodynamics, it might be necessary to tailor drug dosages according to sex and gender.

Certain medications could lead to distinct adverse effects or risks in males and females. An analysis of FDA-approved drugs revealed significant gender-related discrepancies in pharmacokinetics, with the majority of the 86 studied drugs resulting in higher blood concentrations and extended elimination times in women [12]. At the same time, these gender-based pharmacokinetic differences were associated with sex-related adverse drug reactions [12].

12.4 Disease- and Sex-Related Treatment

Gender is an important factor that affects the course of critical illness, but clinical trials have often included more male participants than female ones. This lack of equal gender representation can lead to significant consequences, as explained in the work of Goldstein et al. [13]. Evident gender-based disparities exist in patterns of admission to intensive care units and resource allocation [14]. Although gender can play a crucial role in determining outcomes for critically ill patients, certain factors, such as the impact of sex hormones, remain underexplored.

Gender differences have been noted in the management and outcomes of conditions like ARDS and sepsis. A closer examination of previous studies on ARDS reveals an imbalance in gender representation, with many trials featuring a higher proportion of male participants [15, 16], or lacking mention of sex in baseline characteristics [17]. Secondary analysis from various clinical trials revealed that female patients were less likely to receive lower tidal volume ventilation [18–20], and males exhibited lower driving pressures than females [20]. This is notable, as lower driving pressure is strongly associated with improved survival in ARDS [21].

In sepsis studies, evidence suggests treatment biases, with female patients often experiencing delayed antibiotic therapy compared to males [22, 23]. A retrospective study found that female patients, particularly those under 45 years, were less likely to receive ICU treatment compared to males [14].

Given this, educational curricula should be revised to incorporate new knowledge and enhance training outcomes in gender medicine.

12.5 Research and Data Analysis

Collecting and analyzing sex-disaggregated data in research and clinical practice is a vital step for evidence-based decision-making.

Historically, clinical research was largely skewed toward male participants, disregarding the proper representation of females. This disparity extended to preclinical research involving animal and cell models, which now profoundly affect our comprehension of human biology and disease [24]. The insights gained from such gender-selective research were frequently extrapolated universally, thereby influencing medical treatments to neglect gender differences.

12.5.1 Clinical Research

This systemic exclusion of females, as well as the oversight of transgender, intersex, and individuals with differences of sex development at all stages of research, has created substantial gaps in medical knowledge [25, 26]. This lack of information has consequences on the quality of patient care, leading to diagnostic delays or even incorrect diagnoses, particularly among female patients.

Inadequate representation of women in clinical studies, combined with the absence of gender-based data analysis, has resulted in medications that exhibit diminished efficacy and heightened toxicity among female patients [27]. This imbalance in research representation has implications for healthcare outcomes, highlighting the need for a more inclusive approach to medical research and treatment development.

12.5.2 Preclinical Research

Preclinical studies should include sex-specific data from animal and cell models that account for the biological differences between males and females. This data is essential for understanding how biological sex affects disease progression, treatment response, drug metabolism, and overall health [28]. In preclinical animal studies, particularly those testing new treatments, the inclusion of both sexes is mandatory.

The following principles should be considered in medical training and research:

- Inclusive experimental design: Include both male and female subjects to capture sex-based variations in disease progression, drug responses, and key parameters.
- Sex-specific biomarkers and endpoints: Use these to distinguish male and female responses to treatments.
- Hormonal differences: Integrate sex-based hormonal differences in research and treatment.
- Genetic and epigenetic factors: Analyze sex-specific genetic and epigenetic contributions to disease susceptibility and treatment effects.
- Biological mechanisms: Explore mechanisms underlying sex-related disparities in disease progression and treatment responses.

12.6 Ethical and Sociocultural Considerations

Ethical and sociocultural considerations play a key role in critical care and medicine, affecting decision-making and treatment choices. Healthcare teams need to be prepared to address cultural norms, gender roles, and psychosocial factors that affect patient experiences and preferences. It is important to discuss ethical challenges and gender equity to ensure that care respects patients' values, backgrounds, and autonomy.

To foster an environment of inclusivity and respect, integrating ***cultural competency training*** into curricula is necessary. This integration shall ensure that healthcare providers understand and respect the diverse backgrounds and gender identities of their patients and the resulting consequences for medical care. A relevant study on gender education for medical and nursing students raises concerns about whether healthcare professionals fully understand gender-related concepts [29]. The study highlights areas such as sexism, gender awareness, and sexual harassment as central themes within the discourse of gender equity [29].

Within the critical care and perioperative medicine curricula, the following ethical and sociocultural competences should be considered and addressed:

- *Informed consent:* Healthcare providers must offer clear, culturally sensitive information about the procedure, risks, benefits, and alternatives respecting a patient's right to make informed decisions about their treatment.
- *Health disparities*: Efforts should focus on ensuring equitable access to medical care, addressing ethical concerns related to health disparities based on gender, race, ethnicity, or socioeconomic status.
- *Religious beliefs*: Patients may have religious beliefs that impact their decisions on anesthesia, surgery, blood transfusions, or other treatments. Healthcare pro-

viders should be able to engage in open discussions to understand and respect these beliefs while prioritizing patient safety.

- *Family involvement*: In some cultures, family members play a significant role in medical decisions. It is necessary to respect family members as decision-makers.
- *Language barriers*: Involvement of interpreters or providing translated materials helps patients to fully understand the planned procedures and overcome barriers for clear communication for obtaining informed consent and delivering proper care.
- *Privacy and confidentiality*: Fundamental ethical principles such as patients' privacy and confidentiality must be handled accordingly.
- *Decision-making capacity*: Healthcare providers must be able to assess a patient's decision-making capacity to determine if patients can understand the information provided.
- *Patient autonomy*: Patients are empowered to actively participate in decisions about their health regarding their autonomy, values, preferences, and treatment goals.
- *Vulnerable populations:* Healthcare professionals must pay special attention to vulnerable populations such as minors, elderly individuals, or those with cognitive impairments, to ensure that their rights and well-being are protected.
- *End-of-life care*: When discussing advance directives, resuscitation preferences, and end-of-life care cultural and religious beliefs should be respected and discussed with sensitivity.
- *Shared decision-making*: Collaborative decision-making involves not only patients, but also their families in interaction with healthcare providers. A care plan collaboratively developed respecting the patient's values and preferences is most helpful.
- *Cultural competency*: Healthcare professionals should be aware of and respect the cultural beliefs, practices, and preferences of diverse patient populations. Cultural competency ensures that care is provided in a manner that aligns with each patient's cultural values and norms. The effectiveness of cultural competency training for healthcare providers has been repeatedly demonstrated [30, 31], also in the setting of training for medical students [32].

Addressing ethical and sociocultural considerations in perioperative and critical care medicine promotes patient-centred care, enhances patient satisfaction, and upholds the principles of respect, dignity, and justice. Healthcare providers should **receive training and support** to navigate these complex aspects effectively.

12.7 Communication Skills, Including Inclusive Language

Effective communication skills in critical care and perioperative medicine promoting gender equity ensure that patients across all gender identities receive equitable and respectful treatment. Gender-sensitive communication can enhance patient outcomes, satisfaction, and trust.

Inclusive language refers to using words and expressions that do not isolate specific groups of people. It should encompass attributes of respect, accuracy, impartiality, and alignment with the choices of the individuals and communities under discussion. The AMA Manual of Style highlights important aspects for editors and authors, which, of course, applies to spoken language [33].

Inclusive language is employed to acknowledge diverse gender identities with the aim that transgender and non-binary patients are treated equally and with respect and that their needs are accommodated, including the use of their names and pronouns. Doctors with a lack of language training or awareness might stigmatize minorities in conversation [34, 35].

Reflection Point How confident are you in using terms that respect diverse gender identities, ensuring that transgender and non-binary patients are treated with equality and respect? Consider how the use of appropriate names and pronouns can help create a more inclusive environment. How might a lack of language awareness or training affect your interactions and contribute to stigmatization of minority groups in clinical settings?

Patients' decisions must be valued irrespective of their gender, and healthcare providers should demonstrate genuine empathy and sensitivity to gender-related concerns, acknowledging the potential impact of gender on health experiences.

In this context, it is important to understand how cultural norms and gender roles may influence patients' communication preferences and healthcare decisions. Family dynamics should be respected, with attention given to diverse family structures and roles, involving family members appropriately in discussions and decision-making processes.

Healthcare providers, with every team member being encouraged to advocate for equitable treatment and resources for all patients, should inform patients about gender-specific treatment options and potential side effects.

It has been shown that even a minor change in the content of a medical school curriculum by including transgender medicine significantly increased the students' self-reported willingness to care for transgender patients [36]. This highlights the importance of including such training into curricula for healthcare professionals.

Implicit bias, including ethnic, gender, weight, and age bias, is similarly common among healthcare providers as in the general population and is associated with a lower level of care [37]. Therefore, gender-related biases or disparities encountered should be openly discussed within the healthcare team.

12.8 Continuous Education with Assessment and Feedback

Continuous education, assessment, and feedback form indispensable pillars aiming at healthcare professionals to continually advance their understanding of gender-related issues and refining their practices to provide equitable care for all patients.

Continuous education may include specific workshops, seminars, grand rounds, or webinars that focus on gender equity, cultural sensitivity, and inclusive healthcare practices in critical care and perioperative medicine. An initial step is to raise awareness about the gender imbalance in medicine [38]. Additionally, offering online courses covering diverse topics such as gender-sensitive communication, transgender healthcare, and strategies to address health disparities proves invaluable. Journal clubs focused on gender equity articles catalyze critical analysis and reflective discussions on this subject.

Healthcare providers are encouraged to undergo external assessments that include questions related to gender equity and inclusive care in exams, and certification and application processes. Accurate self-assessment of physicians appears to be insufficient [39]. Clinical observations that evaluate healthcare providers' interactions with patients to assess their gender-sensitive communication and practices can serve as valuable tools.

Finally, the feedback culture is essential, encompassing both peer and patient feedback. The patient feedback can be gathered through surveys or interviews to understand their experiences and perceptions. Guidance and feedback from supervisors or mentors on communication skills and practices are equally essential and must be implemented into the team.

12.9 Faculty Development

Despite an increased awareness of gender and sexual bias in the workplace [40], women remain significantly underrepresented in faculty and leadership roles within critical care and perioperative medicine [41, 42]. Faculty development stands as a critical pathway to fostering gender equity within educational and professional domains. It involves providing comprehensive training, support, and resources to educators and faculty members, enriching their understanding of gender-related issues, refining teaching practices, and cultivating inclusive environments.

Several key components ***contribute to effective faculty development*** for promoting gender equity:

- *Gender sensitivity training:* Conducting workshops and seminars that address gender biases, stereotypes, and inequalities equips faculty members with the tools to recognize and mitigate bias.
- *Inclusive pedagogy:* Inclusive pedagogy plays a pivotal role in equipping educators to integrate teaching strategies that cater to diverse gender identities and learning styles. Research shows that implementing inclusive pedagogical approaches effectively reduces academic outcome gaps [43]. Central aspects of inclusive pedagogy include fostering respect, empathy, active communication, and providing ongoing feedback [44]. Linguistic practices profoundly influence inclusivity, contributing to the inclusion or exclusion of minority groups [45]. Therefore, integrating inclusive language, diverse examples, and varied assessment methods stands as a crucial endeavor within faculty development programs.
- *Implicit bias training:* Implicit bias, or unconscious bias, denotes a predisposition for or against individuals or specific groups. Within healthcare, numerous implicit biases persist, significantly impacting patient outcomes and the interactions among healthcare professionals [46, 47]. Implicit bias training stands as an important intervention to equip faculty members in recognizing, comprehending, and mitigating these unconscious biases that influence their interactions with students, colleagues, and patients. Research indicates that even a single educational session is effective in mitigating implicit biases within academic medicine [48], though the impact on explicit biases remains less pronounced. Such training aims to enhance awareness and understanding of biases, fostering a more equitable and inclusive environment within healthcare and educational settings.
- *Behavioral guidelines and zero discrimination tolerance*: A distressing reality persists wherein many women and individuals within the sexual and gender diverse population encounter discrimination and sexual harassment in critical care and perioperative medicine settings [38, 49].

Despite recognition of the fact that diversity can mitigate disparities and enhance healthcare outcomes for minority groups, women and underrepresented minorities continue to hold fewer positions in academia and leadership roles [50, 51]. Addressing these persistent challenges necessitates the establishment of behavioral guidelines [52] or a zero-tolerance policy toward discrimination and prejudice within these professional domains [53]. Implementing such a policy represents a critical step toward fostering inclusivity, respect, and equitable opportunities within critical care and perioperative medicine settings.

By investing in faculty development initiatives focusing on gender equity, educational institutions can create a more inclusive and supportive environment, allowing all individuals to thrive and reach their full potential, regardless of their sex, race, or gender identity.

Action Points

- Include sex-based differences in anatomy, physiology, pharmacology, and clinical medicine in the existing curricula for perioperative and critical care medicine.
- Implement continuous medical education for healthcare professionals, including training on communication skills and inclusive language, to improve practices and provide equitable care for all patients.
- Make implicit bias training a mandatory part of faculty development to foster a more inclusive and unbiased healthcare environment.

Contributions All authors contributed to the design, data collection, and writing of the manuscript.

Disclosure Regarding recommendations of the sub-chapters 'Research and data analysis' and 'Ethical and sociocultural considerations', generative artificial intelligence (ChatGPT) was used for content generation to assist the authors.

References

1. Blair ML. Sex-based differences in physiology: what should we teach in the medical curriculum? Adv Physiol Educ. 2007;31(1):23–5.
2. Kittnar O. Sex related differences in electrocardiography. Physiol Res. 2023;72(Suppl 2):S127–35.
3. Coleman JR, Moore EE, Schmitt L, Hansen K, Dow N, Freeman K, et al. Estradiol provokes hypercoagulability and affects fibrin biology: a mechanistic exploration of sex dimorphisms in coagulation. J Trauma Acute Care Surg. 2023;94(2):179–86.
4. LoMauro A, Aliverti A. Sex differences in respiratory function. Breathe (Sheff). 2018;14(2):131–40. https://doi.org/10.1183/20734735.000318.
5. Taneja V. Sex hormones determine immune response. Front Immunol. 2018;9:1931.
6. Layton AT, Sullivan JC. Recent advances in sex differences in kidney function. Am J Physiol Renal Physiol. 2019;316(2):F328–31. https://doi.org/10.1152/ajprenal.00584.2018.
7. Regitz-Zagrosek V, Seeland U. Sex and gender differences in clinical medicine. Handb Exp Pharmacol. 2012;214:3–22.
8. Farkouh A, Riedl T, Gottardi R, Czejka M, Kautzky-Willer A. Sex-related differences in pharmacokinetics and pharmacodynamics of frequently prescribed drugs: a review of the literature. Adv Ther. 2020;37(2):644–55.
9. Soldin OP, Mattison DR. Sex differences in pharmacokinetics and pharmacodynamics. Clin Pharmacokinet. 2009;48(3):143–57.
10. Filipescu D, Stefan M. Sex and gender differences in anesthesia: relevant also for perioperative safety? Best Pract Res Clin Anaesthesiol. 2021;35(1):141–53.
11. Scandlyn MJ, Stuart EC, Rosengren RJ. Sex-specific differences in CYP450 isoforms in humans. Expert Opin Drug Metab Toxicol. 2008;4(4):413–24.
12. Zucker I, Prendergast BJ. Sex differences in pharmacokinetics predict adverse drug reactions in women. Biol Sex Differ. 2020;11(1):32.
13. Goldstein RH, Walensky RP. Where were the women? Gender parity in clinical trials. N Engl J Med. 2019;381(26):2491–3.

14. Todorov A, Kaufmann F, Arslani K, Haider A, Bengs S, Goliasch G, et al. Gender differences in the provision of intensive care: a Bayesian approach. Intensive Care Med. 2021;47(5):577–87.
15. Acute Respiratory Distress Syndrome Network, Brower RG, Matthay MA, Morris A, Schoenfeld D, Thompson BT, et al. Ventilation with lower tidal volumes as compared with traditional tidal volumes for acute lung injury and the acute respiratory distress syndrome. N Engl J Med. 2000;342(18):1301–8.
16. Guerin C, Reignier J, Richard JC, Beuret P, Gacouin A, Boulain T, et al. Prone positioning in severe acute respiratory distress syndrome. N Engl J Med. 2013;368(23):2159–68.
17. Papazian L, Forel JM, Gacouin A, Penot-Ragon C, Perrin G, Loundou A, et al. Neuromuscular blockers in early acute respiratory distress syndrome. N Engl J Med. 2010;363(12):1107–16.
18. Han S, Martin GS, Maloney JP, Shanholtz C, Barnes KC, Murray S, et al. Short women with severe sepsis-related acute lung injury receive lung protective ventilation less frequently: an observational cohort study. Crit Care. 2011;15(6):R262.
19. Walkey AJ, Wiener RS. Risk factors for underuse of lung-protective ventilation in acute lung injury. J Crit Care. 2012;27(3):323 e321–329.
20. McNicholas BA, Madotto F, Pham T, Rezoagli E, Masterson CH, Horie S, et al. Demographics, management and outcome of females and males with acute respiratory distress syndrome in the LUNG SAFE prospective cohort study. Eur Respir J. 2019;54(4):1900609.
21. Amato MB, Meade MO, Slutsky AS, Brochard L, Costa EL, Schoenfeld DA, et al. Driving pressure and survival in the acute respiratory distress syndrome. N Engl J Med. 2015;372(8):747–55.
22. Madsen TE, Napoli AM. The DISPARITY-II study: delays to antibiotic administration in women with severe sepsis or septic shock. Acad Emerg Med. 2014;21(12):1499–502.
23. Sunden-Cullberg J, Nilsson A, Inghammar M. Sex-based differences in ED management of critically ill patients with sepsis: a nationwide cohort study. Intensive Care Med. 2020;46(4):727–36.
24. Karp NA, Reavey N. Sex bias in preclinical research and an exploration of how to change the status quo. Br J Pharmacol. 2019;176(21):4107–18.
25. Geller SE, Koch AR, Roesch P, Filut A, Hallgren E, Carnes M. The more things change, the more they stay the same: a study to evaluate compliance with inclusion and assessment of women and minorities in randomized controlled trials. Acad Med. 2018;93(4):630–5.
26. Arnegard ME, Whitten LA, Hunter C, Clayton JA. Sex as a biological variable: a 5-year progress report and call to action. J Womens Health (Larchmt). 2020;29(6):858–64.
27. Daitch V, Turjeman A, Poran I, Tau N, Ayalon-Dangur I, Nashashibi J, et al. Underrepresentation of women in randomized controlled trials: a systematic review and meta-analysis. Trials. 2022;23(1):1038.
28. Beery AK, Zucker I. Sex bias in neuroscience and biomedical research. Neurosci Biobehav Rev. 2011;35(3):565–72.
29. Yang HC. What should be taught and what is taught: integrating gender into medical and health professions education for medical and nursing students. Int J Environ Res Public Health. 2020;17(18):6555.
30. Yu H, Flores DD, Bonett S, Bauermeister JA. LGBTQ + cultural competency training for health professionals: a systematic review. BMC Med Educ. 2023;23(1):558.
31. El Achi D, Brown A, Huguenard S, Khan S, Streff H, Nassef S. Perceived impact of ethnocultural competency training on genetic counselors' clinical interactions. J Genet Couns. 2023;33:605.
32. Kelly ML, Parente V, Redmond R, Willis R, Railey K. Development of a curriculum in cultural determinants of health and health disparities. J Natl Med Assoc. 2023;115(4):428–35.
33. Committee AMAMoS. AMA manual of style. 2020.
34. Alpert AB, Scout NFN, Schabath MB, Adams S, Obedin-Maliver J, Safer JD. Gender- and sexual orientation- based inequities: promoting inclusion, visibility, and data accuracy in oncology. Am Soc Clin Oncol Educ Book. 2022;42:1–17.
35. Poteat T, German D, Kerrigan D. Managing uncertainty: a grounded theory of stigma in transgender health care encounters. Soc Sci Med. 2013;84:22–9.

36. Safer JD, Pearce EN. A simple curriculum content change increased medical student comfort with transgender medicine. Endocr Pract. 2013;19(4):633–7.
37. FitzGerald C, Hurst S. Implicit bias in healthcare professionals: a systematic review. BMC Med Ethics. 2017;18(1):19.
38. Bonomo Y, Zundel S, Martin JH. Addressing unconscious bias for female clinical academics. Intern Med J. 2016;46(4):391–3.
39. Davis DA, Mazmanian PE, Fordis M, Van Harrison R, Thorpe KE, Perrier L. Accuracy of physician self-assessment compared with observed measures of competence: a systematic review. JAMA. 2006;296(9):1094–102.
40. Peel JK, Flexman AM, Cygler J, Kirkham KR, Lorello GR. Standing out or fitting in: a latent projective content analysis of discrimination of women and 2SLGBTQ+ anesthesiologists and providers. J Clin Anesth. 2022;80:110884.
41. Venkatesh B, Mehta S, Angus DC, Finfer S, Machado FR, Marshall J, et al. Women in intensive care study: a preliminary assessment of international data on female representation in the ICU physician workforce, leadership and academic positions. Crit Care. 2018;22(1):211.
42. Bosco L, Lorello GR, Flexman AM, Hastie MJ. Women in anaesthesia: a scoping review. Br J Anaesth. 2020;124(3):e134–47.
43. Dewsbury BM, Swanson HJ, Moseman-Valtierra S, Caulkins J. Inclusive and active pedagogies reduce academic outcome gaps and improve long-term performance. PLoS One. 2022;17(6):e0268620.
44. Cotán A, Aguirre A, Morgado B, Melero N. Methodological strategies of faculty members: moving toward inclusive pedagogy in higher education. Sustainability-Basel. 2021;13(6):3031.
45. Sauntson H. Language, sexuality and inclusive pedagogy. Int J Appl Linguist. 2019;29(3):322–40.
46. Rauf I, Hartmann A, Koumtchev A, Khan SA, Kashyap R. Conscious and unconscious bias: the hidden pandemic of biases in healthcare exacerbated by COVID-19. HCA Healthc J Med. 2022;3(3):89–96.
47. Sheffield V, Hartley S, Stansfield RB, Mack M, Blackburn S, Vaughn VM, et al. Gendered expectations: the impact of gender, evaluation language, and clinical setting on resident trainee assessment of faculty performance. J Gen Intern Med. 2022;37(4):714–22.
48. Girod S, Fassiotto M, Grewal D, Ku MC, Sriram N, Nosek BA, et al. Reducing implicit gender leadership bias in academic medicine with an educational intervention. Acad Med. 2016;91(8):1143–50.
49. Venkatesh B, Corke C, Raper R, Pinder M, Stephens D, Joint G, et al. Findings of the bullying, discrimination and sexual harassment survey: response of the College of Intensive Care Medicine. Crit Care Resusc. 2016;18(4):228–9.
50. Toledo P, Duce L, Adams J, Ross VH, Thompson KM, Wong CA. Diversity in the American society of anesthesiologists leadership. Anesth Analg. 2017;124(5):1611–6.
51. Mehta S, Ahluwalia N, Heybati K, Burns KEA, Owais S, Cook DJ, et al. Diversity of authors of publications from the Canadian critical care trials group. Crit Care Med. 2022;50(4):535–42.
52. Kang SK, Kaplan S. Working toward gender diversity and inclusion in medicine: myths and solutions. Lancet. 2019;393(10171):579–86.
53. Noronha B, Fuchs A, Zdravkovic M, Berger-Estilita J. Gender balance in the medical workplace – a snapshot into anesthesia. Trends Anaesth Crit. 2022;43:4–10.

Improving Wellbeing and Reaching Success in Critical Care and Perioperative Medicine

13

Cristina Honorato-Cia, Francesca Rubulotta, and Vojislava Neskovic

Key Points from the Editors

- The wellbeing of healthcare workers entails several components: realization of the full professional potential, fulfilling lifestyle, mental and spiritual health and overall positive experience. It is recognized as essential for delivering high-quality patient care and achieving professional success, particularly in high-pressure fields such as critical care medicine and perioperative medicine.
- The COVID-19 pandemic has amplified awareness of burnout's causes and consequences, necessitating both personal and institutional strategies to recognize and mitigate its effects.
- Implementing comprehensive wellbeing programs, promoting self-care, recognizing symptoms and early signs and fostering a supportive workplace culture are vital steps in preventing burnout and enhancing overall healthcare worker wellbeing.

C. Honorato-Cia
Department of Anaesthesia and Critical Care, Clínica Universidad de Navarra, Pamplona, Spain
e-mail: chonorato@unav.es

F. Rubulotta
Department of Anaesthesia and Critical Care, Ospedale Gaspare Rodolico, Catania, Italy

International Women in Intensive and Critical Care Medicine, iWIN ETS, Catania, Italy
e-mail: francesca.rubulotta@unict.it

V. Neskovic (✉)
Clinic for Anesthesia and Critical Care, Faculty of Medicine MMA, Military Medical Academy, Belgrade, Serbia

V. Neskovic, F. Rubulotta (eds.), *Diversity, Gender Equity and Inclusion in Critical Care and Perioperative Medicine*,
https://doi.org/10.1007/978-3-031-86286-1_13

Main Objectives
After reading this chapter, you will be able to:

1. Identify the multifaceted nature of professional success in perioperative and critical care medicine, emphasizing the crucial link between personal wellbeing—mental, physical, and emotional—and the ability of healthcare workers to effectively care for patients in high-stakes environments.
2. Recognize the prevalence of burnout among women due to factors such as work-life balance and societal expectations in perioperative medicine and critical care.
3. Assess the need for systemic changes in healthcare settings to improve physician wellbeing.

13.1 Introduction

Success is deeply personal, culturally defined, and shaped by environmental factors, practicality, and a sense of purpose [1]. Integral to this concept is wellbeing, which encompasses both mental and physical health and the ability to navigate everyday stressors while remaining aligned with one's core values, as defined by the World Health Organization [1]. However, the question remains: what does professional success truly mean if it comes at the cost of personal balance? Professional fields like perioperative and critical care medicine are high-stakes environments that demand not only technical expertise and physical resilience but also the ability to communicate effectively and make swift decisions. The COVID-19 pandemic has further underscored these challenges, revealing the immense pressure healthcare professionals face. Ultimately, a troubling paradox must be confronted: in the pursuit of providing the best care for others, is there a sacrifice of personal wellbeing?

The near-total absence of internationally shared guidelines, varying competencies, a general lack of preparedness, inconsistent vocabulary, and sometimes dismissive attitudes from ICU staff towards less experienced colleagues—amid a climate of widespread fear—resulted in high turnover rates, burnout syndrome, and numerous career departures post-pandemic caused by harassment [2].

This chapter will focus on these fundamental questions and on strategies to overcome and prevent burnout while preserving individual wellbeing.

13.2 Wellbeing

Wellbeing can be described in various ways. Khan et al. [3] define wellbeing as an active process through which individuals become aware of their circumstances and make conscious choices towards a more fulfilling existence. This process entails several components, namely:

- A conscious, self-directed, and evolving journey towards realizing one's full potential.
- A multidimensional and holistic approach that includes lifestyle, mental and spiritual health, and environmental factors.
- A positive and affirming experience.

The Oxford Dictionary defines success simply as "the accomplishment of an aim or purpose," and what constitutes that "aim or purpose" is subjective to the individual. However, a substantial body of literature—both medical and non-medical—highlights the deep connection between a healthcare worker's personal wellbeing and their professional effectiveness. Physicians are expected to be knowledgeable, skilled, collaborative, and effective communicators, while also embodying traits such as patience, selflessness, respect, and a willingness to learn. Wellbeing is thus a crucial component of success. Without a commitment to continuous improvement, achieving one's goals becomes increasingly challenging. From a professional perspective, success involves not only mastering the necessary competencies to practice but also facilitating academic growth and excelling in leadership roles [4].

> Reflecting on the words of the esteemed nineteenth-century neurologist Nothnagel, who noted, "Only a good man can be a great physician," it becomes clear that a physician must prioritize their own wellbeing to deliver optimal care.

The requirement to be a good person to be a good physician might cause moral distress. In critical care settings, healthcare professionals often face emotionally intense situations and challenging decision-making processes. For instance, assessing a patient's lifestyle choices—such as substance use or involvement in violent incidents—along with navigating end-of-life scenarios can provoke strong emotional responses and moral distress. Research has shown that moral distress is common among healthcare trainees [5]. Difficult and consequential decisions, such as the cessation of therapeutic interventions for patients unlikely to benefit from continued intensive care, are required [5]. These decisions may be perceived as "top-down directives" from unit directors, fostering conflicts and contributing to the attrition of trained personnel who feel overwhelmed by these experiences [6]. Moreover, religious beliefs can create rigidity in the acceptance of decisions guided strictly by clinical prognosis, leading to feelings of powerlessness among healthcare providers [6].

13.3 Burnout Syndrome (BOS)

The term "burnout syndrome" (BOS) has been recognized since the 1970s and is characterized by a range of signs and symptoms indicative of progressive maladaptation in the workplace [2]. BOS is a psychological condition engendered by chronic interpersonal stressors within the workplace.

The three classic symptoms of burnout include:

1. **Exhaustion:** Feelings of being emotionally and physically drained.
2. **Depersonalization:** A sense of detachment or impersonal response towards patients and work.
3. **Reduced Personal Accomplishment:** Feelings of inefficacy and a diminished sense of achievement in one's work.

These definitions are derived from the Maslach Burnout Inventory (MBI), a widely used tool for assessing burnout syndrome that has been in use and validated for over 30 years [7].

The diagnosis of BOS requires the presence of three components: high emotional exhaustion, high depersonalization, and low personal fulfilment [8]. From this definition, workplace well-being is described as *"the absence of burnout and the presence of professional fulfilment"* [9].

The MBI prompts respondents to indicate the frequency of these emotions in their daily practice using a Likert scale; scores above a certain cut-off indicate the presence of BOS syndrome. A survey conducted in 2007 across 189 French ICUs, which included nearly 1000 participants, revealed critical insights, with 46.5% reporting elevated levels of burnout as assessed by the MBI [10]. Furthermore, clinicians from sexual and gender minority (SGM), groups, comprising individuals who identify as lesbian, gay, bisexual, transgender, or queer (LGBTQ, LGBT+), encounter unique workplace stressors. A 2021 survey of U.S. anaesthesiologists identified SGM status as a significant independent risk factor for BOS [11]. Importantly, the severity of patients' medical conditions did not correlate with MBI scores; however, organizational factors within hospital systems did play a pivotal role [11]. Specifically, variables contributing to heightened MBI scores include the frequency of night shifts, the duration since the last break, and dysfunctional workplace relationships marked by conflicts among colleagues. Furthermore, maladaptive personality traits are also associated with increased rates of burnout, as evidenced by a recent study conducted among Italian anaesthetists and intensivists, which identified paranoid, borderline, and passive-aggressive traits as significantly correlated with higher burnout incidence [12]. A similar survey conducted in China, which involved over 1800 intensivists across 30 provinces, revealed that 82.1% of respondents experienced some level of BOS, with 38.8% reporting severe burnout

[13]. Notably, in this survey women were more significantly affected [13]. While marriage appeared to have a protective effect against BOS, the number of children correlated positively with the incidence of BOS. Job satisfaction among Chinese intensivists was identified as a factor that reduces the incidence of BOS. The primary driver for BOS among these physicians was making treatment decisions, which caused emotional fatigue, insomnia, and dizziness or headaches. Chronic sleep disorders, hepatic steatosis, and lumbar disk herniation were common health issues observed among these professionals [13]. BOS undoubtedly affects patient care and overall service quality. Moreover, it exacerbates the existing shortage of personnel in critical care management roles, which are often viewed as offering limited career advancement opportunities and inadequate financial compensation. The Medscape Physician Lifestyle and Happiness Report for 2023 indicates that only 55% of doctors feel somewhat or very happy outside of work, a significant drop from 81% prior to the pandemic. Once among the happiest specialities, critical care and anaesthesia have fallen to the middle-lower ranks in terms of overall happiness [14]. In this 2023 survey, 35% of anaesthesia providers report feeling burned out, and 19% both burned out *and* depressed, against 40% of specialists that report no symptoms [14]. Of them, almost half (42%) say it impacts their daily life significantly; 36% moderately. ***But only 14% sought professional help***.

13.4 Establishing a Foundation for Wellbeing and Success

Since the early 2000s, physician wellbeing has gained increasing attention, with alarming rates of BOS, substance abuse, depression, fatigue, and even suicide reported among anaesthesiologists [7]. This is a well-known fact, and the reasons given are usually the same: problems with renovating licenses, having scope of practice limited, or impact on their reputation in their workplaces. In 2016, an official statement titled *"Burnout Syndrome in Critical Care Healthcare Professionals. A Call for Action"* was jointly prepared and published by the American College of Chest Physicians (CHEST), the American Thoracic Society (ATS), the Society of Critical Care Medicine (SCCM), and the American Association of Critical-Care Nurses (AACN) in their respective professional journals [15]. By 2020, the National Physician Burnout and Suicide Report revealed a 44% burnout rate among intensive care unit (ICU) physicians, compared to 41% among general anaesthesiologists [16, 17]. This situation, combined with chronic sleep deprivation, to the coexistence of depression, anxiety, and burnout syndrome (BOS) among ICU doctors and nurses [18]. In all these percentages, women consistently rank 5–10% higher than men. And this begins early: 6 months into residency, female residents have higher levels of stress and burnout than their male counterparts [19].

In a survey of 9000 US medical specialists, 9% of males and 11% of females had at some point had suicidal thoughts [20]. This is a critical issue with profound implications, particularly regarding the cost in human lives. In the early 2000s, as burnout began to emerge, personal coping strategies were recommended.

Reflection Point The pandemic has made it increasingly clear that healthcare systems rely heavily on their professionals without adequately addressing the root causes of BOS. What are the potential risk factors contributing to the higher incidence of suicide among doctors compared to the general population? Could the over idealization of medical roles and excessively high self-expectations be contributing factors as well?

13.4.1 System-Related Factors Increasing Risk for Burnout

- *Increasing workload*
  The ratio of patients per physician keeps growing, allowing less time to properly performed care, and created a trusting relationship. As the burden of direct patient care shifts to allied professionals, physicians lose the personal gratification that comes from building meaningful relationships with patients. In turn, patients are reduced to numbers rather than individuals with unique stories and goals, leading to a perception of lower-quality care [19]. Moreover, the increased reliance on allied professions and stricter regulatory practices have led to the implementation of rigid protocols and policies. While these are essential for ensuring patient safety, they may not always be recognized by the professionals as the patient's best interest moving away from individualized medicine. Meeting patients' demands becomes impossible due to the lack of flexibility and control over schedules that many physicians face. The growing work pressure is a significant stressor, contributing to BOS and depression among healthcare professionals [20]. This not only affects patient care: 55% of female anaesthesiologists report feeling conflicted about balancing their roles as parents, compared to 33% of their male counterparts [14]. Explaining this result and the correlation between anxiety, depression, wellbeing, and performance in ICU is complex [6]. There is also scarcity of scientific literature focusing on healthcare workers' perspectives regarding discrimination, workplace violence, and wellbeing. The authors will discuss these matters in more detail in the next chapter.
- *Increasing bureaucracy*
  Adding to all the previous issues, more documentation needs to be undertaken, often through rigid electronic medical records. Obtaining information from other hospitals (that operate with different electronic systems) can be as stressful. Trainees had to spend long hours in front of electronic medical record [21]. It's no secret that doctors spend increasing amounts of time in front of computers rather than patients. Hansen explored the concept "computer vs. patient: Fighting for residents' attention: what does this mean for medical trainees?" [21] Recent research discovered that the trainees spent 5.38 h—or nearly half of a 12-h work day—in front of a screen, on average. This was tracked with prior research from others, conducted through observations and questionnaires. The researchers found that chart review accounted for the largest proportion of computer activity

by all residents, followed by note entry. That meant residents were spending more time looking for information or adding new information compared to visiting patients [21].

- *Lack of clear leadership/institutional policies*
  There is a general perception that systems are difficult to change and that they are not evolving over time. Many of the stressors mentioned before, lie in the system: staffing, work hours, relief systems; inadequate compensation; lack of support for second victims or stressed-out physicians; insufficient diversity or equity support policies. However, in the past 10 years, it has become more apparent that institutional policies recognize more physician wellbeing and burnout rates, both to prevent and to cope with them [22].
- *Social bias*
  The practice environment is influenced by deeply rooted attitudes and preconceptions These biases may contribute to detrimental outcomes for healthcare professionals. Arnold-Forster et al. [23] identify three key aspects that significantly impact wellbeing:

Three key aspects that impact wellbeing:

Medical Exceptionalism: This concept suggests that practicing medicine requires self-sacrifice, which can lead to unhealthy behaviours and unsafe work practices. Consequently, this mindset makes physicians vulnerable to exploitation by the healthcare system, often to the detriment of their own wellbeing.

Medicalization: There is a pervasive belief that physicians who experience mental health or substance abuse issues are unfit to practice. This stigma can deter healthcare professionals from seeking the help they need, exacerbating their struggles.

Shifting the responsibility to individual: This notion places the onus of maintaining wellness solely on the physician. While it is important for physicians to take ownership of their wellbeing, this perspective can excuse employers from making meaningful changes or implementing comprehensive support programs, instead promoting minimal, cost-effective solutions that do not adequately address the needs of medical professionals.

13.4.2 Individual-Related Factors Increasing Risk for Burnout

Individuals, for their part, have some characteristics that make them vulnerable. Some of them are related to personality traits as they influence how stress or display coping options are experienced [24]. Stress is a compound response to perceived threats and consists in a set of endocrine, immunological, behavioural, cognitive and emotional reactions, all happening very rapidly and synchronically.

Specifically, production of cortisol and changes in the function of the hypothalamic-pituitary-adrenal axis are well known to happen when exposed to chronic stress. Both the locus coeruleus and the dorsal raphe seem to be involved in the modulation of the stress response and are the site of the opioids versus CRF (corticotropin-releasing factor) action. CRF is thought to be the main neuromodulator involved in coordinating the autonomic and behavioural response to stress [25]. In this context, individual variations in genetic expression, receptor sensitivity, and polymorphisms explain why people experience different levels of distress and suffer varying consequences. Research indicates that women possess lower mu-opioid receptor sensitivity than men, correlating with the higher prevalence of stress-related diseases among women [25]. Additionally, individuals with higher neuroticism—a personality trait characterized by a tendency to experience negative emotions such as anger, anxiety, or sadness—are more prone to elevated stress levels and a sense of hopelessness, making them likely candidates for burnout [26]. Such individuals often endure physical symptoms, including headaches, fatigue, and abdominal pain [27]. Further, past negative experiences, inadequate social support (especially given that anaesthetists and intensivists frequently work antisocial hours), and poor coping skills present significant barriers to wellbeing [27, 28].

Reflection Point A term that encapsulates the capacity to overcome these challenges is resilience. Defined as "the ability to recover from or adjust easily to misfortune or change," resilience has gained recognition in recent years as a crucial component of physician wellness. Various resources and institutional programs now aim to foster resilience through training and workshops. Can you quote a time when resilience was needed in your career?

While resilience is important, it mainly focuses on the individual. Teaching doctors just to cope with stress isn't enough to remediate systemic problems [28]. Physicians should prioritize their own wellbeing, while healthcare managers must make systemic changes to support the wellbeing of their staff. Organizations must actively work to improve practices that promote the health of healthcare professionals. The balance between compassion fatigue (negative elements) and compassion satisfaction (positive elements) forms the basis for scoring systems like the Professional Quality of Life (ProQOL), validated by Stamm and colleagues [29]. Research indicates compassion fatigue and BOS are more prevalent among ICU nurses than ICU physicians, possibly due to the current nationwide nursing shortage. Moreover, practicing in ICU and perioperative medicine can be psychologically challenging for ICU residents encountering such demanding environments for the first time [28]. Although stress and anxiety are common among anaesthesia residents, a recent small-scale single-centre experience demonstrated that cognitive performance, as measured by the 'revised' Tower of London Test (TOL-R), improved after day shift in ICU residents, although the improvement was less pronounced in the context of intraoperative emergencies [30] (Table 13.1).

Table 13.1 System and individual factors related to burnout

System-related	Individual-related
Increasing workload Excessive bureaucracy Lack of clear leadership or goals Poor work organization and provision of resting times Lack of clinical autonomy or recognition Antisocial hours, on call Health and wellness being nonpriority	Female gender Seniority: Residents—Younger specialists Predisposing personality traits (neuroticism, perfectionism) Poor social network at work, at home, or both Communication difficulties affecting conflict with other professionals Moral distress Compassion fatigue

13.5 Burnout, the Main Obstacle to Physician Wellness and Success

It is important to recognize that comparing BOS across different professions presents challenges, including establishing appropriate cut-off values specific to each field [31, 32]. This distinction is significant because the loss of empathy, a common consequence of BOS, can have potentially severe implications, particularly in healthcare settings, where interpersonal relationships and emotional connections with patients are vital for effective care [32]. The MBI is used to identify BOS alongside the Areas of Work life Survey (AWS), which assesses various factors affecting job satisfaction, including workload, job demands, efficiency, resource availability, control and flexibility, work-life balance, social support both at work and outside, recognition, and alignment with personal values [33]. A variation of this AWS has been implemented by the Society of Critical Care Medicine as an assessment tool specifically designed for Intensive Care Units [28].

> The boundaries between burnout syndrome (BOS) and depression can sometimes be indistinct [19], increasing the associated risks of each condition. As discussed earlier, burnout can progress to severe outcomes, including suicidal ideation.

Other overlapping conditions include compassion fatigue, moral distress, and perceptions of inadequate patient care.

- Moral Distress: This occurs when practitioners are aware of the right course of action but find themselves in situations that make it nearly impossible to act accordingly [34]. Contributing factors include self-doubt, environmental constraints, limited access to necessary techniques or medications, inadequate training, and lack of communication or viable solutions due to power dynamics. Recent surveys indicate that ICU nurses experience moral distress more frequently than doctors [18], with women showing a higher prevalence than men.

- Inappropriate Patient Care: This can arise from situations marked by excessive workload, perceived futility of aggressive treatment, inadequate quality of care, or the dismissal of a patient's wishes [6].
- Compassion Fatigue: This term describes the gradual decline in one's compassion over time, driven by increasing frustrations within the practitioner's environment. Studies report that up to 25% of ICU nurses and 32% of ICU physicians experience compassion fatigue [29].

13.6 Women and Burnout

Unsurprisingly, women experience a high prevalence of burnout from the early stages of their careers. Within just 6 months of residency, female residents report higher levels of stress and burnout compared to their male counterparts [4, 29]. Some studies suggest that women are more likely to exhibit outward symptoms of burnout, scoring higher in emotional exhaustion, while men tend to show greater levels of depersonalization [34]. A recent review by Klick et al. on Critical Care physicians indicates that burnout rates average around 40% across various sources in Europe and North America, with a significant post-pandemic spike in anxiety scores, reaching up to 60% overall and 73% in women [35].

Although factors such as age, specialty, practice type, and personality can influence burnout rates, it is evident that women and men experience burnout differently. External factors affecting both genders have varied impacts; for instance, work-life integration is notably cited more often by women as a significant contributor, while issues such as gender discrimination and harassment also rank highly [36].

A study by Cardador et al. demonstrates that women surgeons encounter workplace harassment more frequently than their male counterparts, facing behaviours or requests that are often overlooked for male surgeons, especially among nurses and ancillary staff [37]. Cultural expectations also play a role, particularly the perception of women as caregivers, which can influence physician-patient relationships. Women are documented to spend more time in patient visits and to explore socio-emotional and psychosocial issues more thoroughly [36]. The stereotype of the "motherly doctor" can increase the likelihood of burnout, particularly in the realm of compassion fatigue, affecting all medical specialities. Burnout manifests differently in everyone, leading to distinct "subtypes" of burnout, as described by Maslach and Leiter in a recent Harvard Business Review article [38]. Understanding these variations is crucial, as both the consequences of burnout and the strategies to address them will differ accordingly.

Burnout syndrome is characterized by negative scores in exhaustion, cynicism, and perceptions of professional efficacy. Possible subvariants include overextended burnout (where individuals score disproportionately high in emotional exhaustion), ineffective burnout (related to perceived inefficacy), and disengaged burnout (where cynicism predominates). **Women are more likely to experience overextended or disengaged burnout,** leading to different consequences and coping mechanisms.

13.7 The Consequences of Burnout

Reduced efficiency and productivity are two major external consequences of burnout. Furthermore, the risks of depression, substance abuse, and suicide escalate significantly, each carrying a heavy human cost [33]. The impact of burnout extends beyond physicians; families, patients, and entire communities bear the repercussions of a healthcare worker's burnout [39].

Reduced productivity in healthcare leads to staffing challenges, with higher absenteeism and presenteeism—where doctors are physically present but too overextended to be effective. Academic clinicians also report lower engagement with students, reduced teaching quality, and decreased confidence in their own learning. As a result, many physicians change hospitals more often or even consider leaving the profession [40, 41].

Doctor-patient relationships are significantly impacted by compassion fatigue, which diminishes physicians' empathy and patience. This fatigue can lead to **miscommunications** with patients and their families and **reduce situational awareness during critical interactions**.

The consequences of burnout are listed in Table 13.2.

Table 13.2 Consequences of burnout [42]

Patient care	Deterioration of relationships (doctor-patient and doctor-other professionals). Increased medical errors and malpractice. Lower patient satisfaction. Lower overall quality of care and outcomes.
Health care cost	Higher physician turnover. Physicians leaving the profession. Increase in time, effort, and money involved in recruitment and training. Higher risk of legal claims and associated costs.
Physician health	Frequent complaints of feeling tired, exhausted, fatigued, inattentive, and irritable. Increased risk of motor vehicle accidents and near-miss events, even after adjusting for fatigue. Reports of feeling stressed, disruptive behaviour, mood disorders, and depression. Higher incidence of substance abuse, and in surgical specialities, abuse or dependence on alcohol. Increased risk of suicidal ideation.

13.8 Addressing Burnout: Prevention and Promotion of Wellbeing

Fostering wellbeing encompasses more than just preventing burnout and many strategies are interconnected. The following approaches will be presented collectively, outlining strategies that can be applied to various circumstances and workplace settings to promote wellbeing and prevent burnout.

13.8.1 Individual Measures

Following strategies are widely recognized, it is important to emphasize that they are not only well-established through experience but also supported by scientific evidence [43].

- Mindfulness and other relaxation and acceptance training techniques. Sessions as short as 20 minutes in three consecutive days have shown positive results in wellbeing, but there are many resources including apps that can help busy healthcare workers.
- Continued physical activity, within adequate limits.
- Healthy nutrition and sleep schedules (this can be difficult sometimes but should at least be preserved during adequately scheduled breaks and vacations).
- Promoting and engaging in a supportive work environment, where peer support is the norm and not the exception.
- Spending time with family and friends.
- Having a person (or a circle of persons) where venting can be done safely when needed.
- Choosing fulfilling hobbies and extracurricular activities.

13.8.2 Organizational Strategies

There is an increased awareness of the necessity of addressing burnout and its consequences from an institutional, systematic, and professional perspective. As stated before, healthcare workers are often expected to take care of themselves to stay mentally and physically fit and healthy, but this approach is often unreliable and is fundamentally unfair; the wellbeing of healthcare providers impacts directly the whole community.

As a prime example, the European Parliament issued the 2021 European Union Directive on work-life balance for parents and caregivers, aimed at fostering a better equilibrium between family and professional commitments while providing equal opportunities for women and men in both the workplace and at home [44]. Key provisions of the directive include extended maternity and paternity leave, leave for caregivers, the right to request flexible working arrangements, and protection against dismissal related to these circumstances. Implementation of the directive varies across countries, as while they are required to comply, the resources allocated for its execution may differ. The European Network for Work-Life Balance (ENWLB) and the European Agency for Safety and Health at Work (EU-OSHA) are among agencies that offer a range of resources, including research, training materials, and best practices available on their websites.

Professional associations have developed a range of resources to address burnout, recognizing its impact and the specific challenges it poses for their members.

- The **European Society of Anesthesiology and Intensive Care Medicine (ESAIC)** and the **American Society of Anesthesiologists (ASA)** both feature dedicated sections on burnout that encompass its causes, symptoms, and prevention tips.
- The **Society of Critical Care Medicine (SCCM)** provides information on burnout through its website, including a self-assessment tool.
- National critical care medicine, intensive care medicine, and anaesthesiology societies also produce guidance documents on the topic and have contributed to national or international directives addressing this issue. For example, in the United Kingdom, the **National Institute for Health and Care Excellence (NICE)** has developed related guidelines.

These resources can assist in tailoring policies to fit the unique characteristics and needs of specific departments or hospitals. While the final endorsement and implementation of such policies will come from hospital and departmental management, anaesthesiology and critical care staff play a crucial role in recognizing their colleagues at risk and offering support. They are also well-placed to promote workplace changes that enhance working conditions—such as optimizing workflow, improving the physical environment, creating flexible arrangements, and fostering a more meaningful care experience. This proactive approach addresses burnout before it occurs, rather than solely focusing on treatment.

> To promote wellbeing among healthcare workers at the hospital level, several strategies can be implemented: ensuring adequate staffing levels, providing opportunities for professional development and support, encouraging regular breaks and vacations, and establishing programs that enhance work-life balance.

It is essential to recognize that while self-care resources can be beneficial, ***they cannot replace professional medical assistance when clear signs of burnout are present.*** A culture of mutual support within the medical community is necessary. It requires providing genuine support, refraining from negative comments, and acknowledging the significant changes in the workplace. By fostering such an environment, the likelihood of burnout can be significantly reduced.

13.9 Balancing Professional Success and Personal Wellbeing

Success is a complex and multifaceted concept, shaped by various perspectives and influences. Achieving true success requires a holistic approach, where academic achievement is balanced with a personal sense of purpose, fostering growth both individually and within one's environment. This is particularly important for women, who often face societal pressures to "have it all," often at a significant personal cost.

The responsibility for creating a functional and compassionate work culture lies with everyone. This culture should minimize obstacles and ensure reasonable, supportive expectations for all individuals. Both leaders and non-leaders must contribute to this effort. The culture established today will shape future generations, fostering an environment that promotes excellence, wellbeing, and support, ultimately leading to a sense of personal achievement and purpose.

13.10 Lesson Learnt from COVID-19

The absence of clear guidelines and a lack of preparedness led to rising tensions, increased workloads, and ineffective communication [2]. The shortage of personal protective equipment (PPE) further exacerbated fears among CCM workers about potentially infecting their families, significantly contributing to the worsening of BOS and anxiety [2, 45]. The fear and uncertainty surrounding the pandemic exacerbated these dynamics, leading to a toxic workplace culture where frustration and stress could manifest as interpersonal conflicts [45]. The isolation experienced by healthcare workers—stemming from fears of transmitting the virus to family members and a shortage of resources—further hindered the development of supportive relationships among team members, leaving many feelings marginalized. Establishing a culture of respect and support is crucial for protecting the mental health and safety of all healthcare professionals, especially in times of crisis. A review conducted in ICUs during the pandemic identified significant challenges in managing the home-work interface. The increased workload, compounded by the contraction of welfare services—such as the closure of childcare facilities—made it extremely difficult for staff to balance their professional and personal lives [46]. The risk of transmitting the virus to family members and the PPE shortages led healthcare workers to become isolated, making communication more challenging and increasing the risk of burnout [47]. The World Health Organization (WHO) estimates that approximately 179,500 healthcare workers (HCWs) died globally because of the pandemic. Initially lauded as "heroes" by the media and politicians during the crisis, staff often found themselves neither financially rewarded nor professionally recognized [48]. During the vaccine rollout phase, widespread scepticism among the public also affected healthcare workers (HCWs), leading to increased tensions and potential harassment within the workforce [45]. Many HCWs, despite their knowledge and exposure to the virus, refused vaccination due to concerns about side effects. This resulted in suspensions or dismissals, creating an environment of fear and discrimination against those with differing beliefs [49].

According to Fessell et al. [50], the major risk factors for burnout syndrome (BOS) during the pandemic can be categorized as follows:

1. Personal Characteristics: Traits such as self-criticism, idealism, perfectionism, inadequate coping strategies, sleep deprivation, and excessive overcommitment [28].
2. Organizational Factors: Issues including unmanageable workloads, a lack of autonomy over the work environment, insufficient rewards, and a general breakdown of workplace community [19].
3. Quality of Working Relationships: Conflicts among multidisciplinary teams tasked with the care of complex patients.
4. Exposure to End-of-Life Issues: Critical care nurses reported heightened burnout levels associated with providing care for dying patients, witnessing end-of-life transitions, and participating in comfort care protocols.

Furthermore, the pandemic exacerbated unprecedented anxiety and conflicts among intensivists, driven by resource shortages and the enforcement of mandatory preventative measures, such as mask-wearing, social distancing, minimizing superspreader events, and vaccination to mitigate severe illness [51]. Such conditions severely undermined workplace wellbeing. Nevertheless, valuable insights were gained regarding ICU wellbeing during and after the pandemic. The Royal College of Anaesthetists summarized the "10 lessons learned from COVID-19" (https://www.rcoa.ac.uk/policy/policy-public-affairs/covid-19-campaign/10-lessons-learnt-covid-19), highlighting key points [52].

Action Points

- Create structured support networks, in critical care and perioperative medicine. This can provide a platform for sharing experiences, coping strategies, and resources to help deal with stress and burnout.
- Develop comprehensive wellbeing initiatives that focus on mental health, stress management, and work-life balance. Include regular training sessions on resilience, mindfulness practices, and access to counselling services in high-pressure environments.
- Create an environment of trust and openness towards mental health problems in critical care and anaesthesia. Make professional help available for those in need.

References

1. WHO. Thirteenth General Programme of Work 2019–2023. 2018. Available from: https://apps.who.int/iris/bitstream/handle/10665/324775/WHO-PRP-18.1-eng.pdf
2. Feeley T, Ffrench-O'Carroll R, Tan MH, Magner C, L'Estrange K, O'Rathallaigh E, Whelan S, Lyons B, O'Connor E. A model for occupational stress amongst paediatric and adult critical care staff during COVID-19 pandemic. Int Arch Occup Environ Health. 2021;94(7):1721–37.
3. Khan A, Vinson AE. Physician well-being in practice. Anesth Analg [Internet]. 2020 Nov 1 [cited 2023 Aug 25];131(5):1359–69. Available from: https://journals.lww.com/anesthesia-analgesia/fulltext/2020/11000/physician_well_being_in_practice.8.aspx
4. Rizo CA, Jadad AR, Enkin M. What's a good doctor and how do you make one?: doctors should be good companions for people. Br Med J [Internet] 2002 Sep 9 [cited 2023 Aug 27];325(7366):711. Available from: /pmc/articles/PMC1124230/.
5. Piers RD, Azoulay E, Ricou B, et al. Appropricus Study Group of the Ethics Section of the European Society of Intensive Care Medicine. Inappropriate care in European ICUs: confronting views from nurses and junior and senior physicians. Chest. 2014;146(2):267–75. https://doi.org/10.1378/chest.14-0256.
6. Azoulay E, Timsit JF, Sprung CL, et al. Conflicus study investigators and for the ethics section of the European Society of Intensive Care Medicine. Prevalence and factors of intensive care unit conflicts: the conflicus study. Am J Respir Crit Care Med. 2009;180(9):853–60. https://doi.org/10.1164/rccm.200810-1614OC.
7. World Health Organization. The impact of COVID-19 on health and care workers: a closer look at deaths. World Health Organization (2021). https://iris.who.int/handle/10665/345300
8. Kira IA, Shuwiekh HAM, Ashby JS, Elwakeel SA, Alhuwailah A, Sous MSF, Baali SBA, Azdaou C, Oliemat EM, Jamil HJ. The impact of COVID-19 traumatic stressors on mental health: is COVID-19 a new trauma type. Int J Ment Health Addict. 2023;21(1):51–70.
9. Stobbs C. Maintaining personal resilience in this Covid-19 era. In Pract. 2021;43(2):109–12.
10. Embriaco N, Azoulay E, Barrau K, Kentish N, Pochard F, Loundou A, Papazian L. High level of burnout in intensivists: prevalence and associated factors. Am J Respir Crit Care Med. 2007;175(7):686–92.
11. Afonso AM, Cadwell JB, Staffa SJ, Zurakowski D, Vinson AE. Burnout rate and risk factors among anesthesiologists in the United States. Anesthesiology. 2021;134(5):683–96. https://doi.org/10.1097/ALN.0000000000003722.
12. Vittori A, Petrucci E, Cascella M, Bignami EG, Simonini A, Sollecchia G, Fiore G, Vergallo A, Marinangeli F, Pedone R. Maladaptive personality traits are associated with burnout risk in

Italian anesthesiologists and intensivists: a secondary analysis from a cross-sectional study. J Anesth Analg Crit Care. 2024;4(1):36.
13. Wang J, Hu B, Peng Z, Song H, Cai S, Rao X, Li L, Li J. Prevalence of burnout among intensivists in mainland China: a nationwide cross-sectional survey. Crit Care. 2021;25(1):8.
14. https://www.medscape.com/sites/public/lifestyle/2023
15. Moss M, Good VS, Gozal D, Kleinpell R, Sessler CN. A critical care societies collaborative statement: burnout syndrome in critical care health-care professionals. A call for action. Am J Respir Crit Care Med. 2016;194(1):106–13.
16. Pines A, Maslach C. Characteristics of staff burnout in mental health settings. Hosp Community Psychiatry. 1978;29(4):233–7.
17. Leslie Kane MA. Medscape National Physician Burnout & Suicide Report 2020: The Generational Divide (2020). https://www.medscape.com/slideshow/2020-lifestyle-burnout-6012460#3 January 15.
18. Mealer M. Burnout syndrome in the intensive care unit. Future directions for research. Ann Am Thorac Soc. 2016;13(7):997–8.
19. Guille C, Frank E, Zhao Z, Kalmbach DA, Nietert PJ, Mata DA, et al. Work-family conflict and the sex difference in depression among training physicians. JAMA Int Med [Internet]. 2017;177(12):1766.
20. https://www.medscape.com/slideshow/2023-family-med-suicide-rpt-6016297?icd=login_success_email_match_norm
21. https://scopeblog.stanford.edu/2019/02/13/computer-vs-patient-fighting-for-residents-attention/
22. Stehman CR, Clark RL, Purpura A, Kellogg AR. Wellness: combating burnout and its consequences in emergency medicine. West J Emerg Med. 2020;21(3):555–65. Published 2020 Apr 13. https://doi.org/10.5811/westjem.2020.1.40971.
23. Arnold-Forster A, Moses JD, Schotland SV. Obstacles to physicians' emotional health — lessons from history. N Engl J Med. 2022;386(1):4–7.
24. Lapa TA, Madeira FM, Viana JS, Pinto-Gouveia J. Burnout syndrome and wellbeing in anesthesiologists: the importance of emotion regulation strategies. Minerva Anestesiol. 2017;83(2):191–9.
25. Tsigos C, Chrousos GP. Hypothalamic-pituitary-adrenal axis, neuroendocrine factors and stress. J Psychosom Res. 2002;53(4):865–71. https://doi.org/10.1016/s0022-3999(02)00429-4. PMID: 12377295
26. Widiger TA, Oltmanns JR. Neuroticism is a fundamental domain of personality with enormous public health implications. World Psychiatry. 2017;16(2):144–5. https://doi.org/10.1002/wps.20411. PMID: 28498583; PMCID: PMC5428182
27. van der Wal RAB, Wallage J, Bucx MJL. Occupational stress, burnout and personality in anesthesiologists. Curr Opin Anaesthesiol. 2018;31(3):351–6.
28. https://www.sccm.org/clinical-resources/well-being-resources
29. Stamm BH. The concise ProQOL manual. 2nd ed. Pocatello: ProQOL.org; 2010.
30. Boscolo A, Queirolo L, Navalesi P. The impact of psychophysiological well being on November 28, 2024. https://doi.org/10.1097/EJA.0000000000002106.
31. https://www.who.int/standards/classifications/frequently-asked-questions/burn-out-an-occupational-phenomenon1
32. Brom SS, Buruck G, Horváth I, et al. Areas of worklife as predictors of occupational health—a validation study in two German samples. Burn Res. 2015;2(2–3):60–70. https://doi.org/10.1016/j.burn.2015.05.001.
33. https://www.mindgarden.com/117-maslach-burnout-inventory-mbi
34. Hinzmann D, Schütte-Nütgen K, Büssing A, Boenisch O, Busch HJ, Dodt C, et al. Critical care providers' moral distress: frequency, burden, and potential resources. Int J Environ Res Public Health. 2023;20(1)
35. Klick JC, Syed M, Leong R, Miranda H, Cotter EK. Health and Well-being of intensive care unit physicians: how to ensure the longevity of a critical specialty. Anesthesiol Clin. 2023;41(1):303–16.

36. Templeton K, Bernstein CA, Sukhera J, Nora LM, Newman C, Burstin H, et al. Gender-based differences in burnout: issues faced by women physicians. NAM Perspectives. 2019;28
37. Cardador MT, Hill PL, Salles A. Unpacking the status-leveling burden for women in male-dominated occupations. Adm Sci Q. 2022;67(1):237–84.
38. Maslach C, Leiter MP. How to measure burnout accurately and ethically. Harv Bus Rev. 2021;
39. Menon NK, Shanafelt TD, Sinsky CA, Linzer M, Carlasare L, Brady KJS, et al. Association of physician burnout with suicidal ideation and medical errors. JAMA Netw Open. 2020;3(12):e2028780.
40. Nassar AK, Waheed A, Tuma F. Academic clinicians' workload challenges and burnout analysis. Cureus. 2019;11(11):e6108.
41. Sinskey JL, Margolis RD, Vinson AE. The wicked problem of physician well-being, Anesthesiology clinics, vol. 40. W.B. Saunders; 2022. p. 213–23.
42. Patel R, Bachu R, Adikey A, Malik M, Shah M. Factors related to physician burnout and its consequences: a review. Behav Sci. 2018;8(11):98.
43. Razai MS, Kooner P, Majeed A. Strategies and interventions to improve healthcare professionals' well-being and reduce burnout. J Prim Care Community Health. 2023;14:21501319231178641. https://doi.org/10.1177/21501319231178641.
44. http://www.inclusion-europe.eu/work-life-balance-directive/
45. Cag Y, Erdem H, Gormez A, Ankarali H, Hargreaves S, Ferreira-Coimbra J, Rubulotta F, Belliato M, Berger-Estilita J, Pelosi P, Blot S, Lefrant JY, Mardani M, Darazam IA, Cag Y, Rello J. Anxiety among front-line health-care workers supporting patients with COVID-19: A global survey. Gen Hosp Psychiatry. 2021;68:90–6. https://doi.org/10.1016/j.genhosppsych.2020.12.010. Epub 2020 Dec 20. PMID: 33418193; PMCID: PMC7749993
46. Gualano MR, Sinigaglia T, Lo Moro G, Rousset S, Cremona A, Bert F, Siliquini R. The burden of burnout among healthcare professionals of intensive care units and emergency departments during the COVID-19 pandemic: a systematic review. Int J Environ Res Public Health. 2021;18(15):8172. https://doi.org/10.3390/ijerph18158172. PMID: 34360465; PMCID: PMC8346023
47. Askarian M, Semenov A, Llopis F, Rubulotta F, Dragovac G, Pshenichnaya N, Assadian O, Ruch Y, Shayan Z, Padilla Fortunatti C, Lucey D, Almohaizeie A, Kamal AHM, Ogunshe A, Konkayev A, Beg A, Primerano E, Amer F, Kumari Pilli HP, Hung I, Ayoade F, Lefrant JY, Zajkowska J, Rello J, Kazi M, Taghrir MH, Blot S, Leib S, Hosseinpour P, Hosseinpour H, Erfani A, Borazjani R, Akbarialiabad H, Najafi M, Askarian A, Erdem H. The COVID-19 vaccination acceptance/hesitancy rate and its determinants among healthcare workers of 91 countries: a multicenter cross-sectional study. EXCLI J. 2022;21:93–103. https://doi.org/10.17179/excli2021-4439. PMID: 35221837; PMCID: PMC8859647
48. World Health Organization. The impact of COVID-19 on health and care workers: a closer look at deaths. World Health Organization (2021). https://iris.who.int/handle/10665/345300.
49. Parodi E. Italy to end ban on health workers not vaccinated against Covid. (2022). https://www.reuters.com/business/healthcare-pharmaceuticals/Italy-end-ban-health-workers-not-vaccinated-against-covid-2022-10-28/ by Reuters October 2022.
50. Fessell D, Cherniss C. Coronavirus disease 2019 (COVID-19) and beyond: micropractices for burnout prevention and emotional wellness. J Am Coll Radiol. 2020;17(6):746–8.
51. Sachs JD, Karim SSA, Aknin L, Allen J, Brosbøl K, Colombo F, Barron GC, Espinosa MF, Gaspar V, Gaviria A, Haines A, Hotez PJ, Koundouri P, Bascuñán FL, Lee JK, Pate MA, Ramos G, Reddy KS, Serageldin I, Thwaites J, Vike-Freiberga V, Wang C, Were MK, Xue L, Bahadur C, Bottazzi ME, Bullen C, Laryea-Adjei G, Ben Amor Y, Karadag O, Lafortune G, Torres E, Barredo L, Bartels JGE, Joshi N, Hellard M, Huynh UK, Khandelwal S, Lazarus JV, Michie S. The lancet commission on lessons for the future from the COVID-19 pandemic. Lancet. 2022;400(10359):1224–80.
52. https://www.rcoa.ac.uk/policy/policy-public-affairs/covid-19-campaign/10-lessons-learnt-covid-19

Preventing Harassment to Improve Team Well-Being and Patient Safety in Healthcare

14

Raffaele Aspide, Ornella Piazza, Marcela Vizcaychipi, Alice Agostinelli, Naeha Geogy, and Deeya Sharma

Abbreviations

ED	Emergency Department
CCM	Critical Care Medicine
CHEST	American College of Chest Physicians
ATS	American Thoracic Society
SCCM	Society of Critical Care Medicine
AACN	American Association of Critical-Care Nurses
ICU	Intensive Care Unit
ESICM	European Society of Intensive Care Medicine
BOS	Burnout syndrome

R. Aspide (✉)
IRCCS Istituto delle Scienze Neurologiche di Bologna – Anesthesia and Intensive Care Unit, Bologna, Italy
e-mail: raffaele.aspide@isnb.it

O. Piazza
Department of Medicine, University of Salerno, Salerno, Italy
e-mail: opiazza@unisa.it

M. Vizcaychipi
Imperial College London, London, UK

Chelsea & Westminster NHS Foundation Trust, London, UK
e-mail: m.vizcaychipi@imperial.ac.uk

A. Agostinelli
Barts and The London School of Medicine and Dentistry, London, UK

N. Geogy · D. Sharma
University of Washington, Seattle, WA, USA
e-mail: naehag@uw.edu

V. Neskovic, F. Rubulotta (eds.), *Diversity, Gender Equity and Inclusion in Critical Care and Perioperative Medicine*,
https://doi.org/10.1007/978-3-031-86286-1_14

ProQOL	Professional Quality of Life
HCWs	healthcare workers
JAMA	The Journal of the American Medical Association
US	United States
PPE	Personal Protective Equipment
WHO	World Health Organization
MBI	Maslach Burnout Inventory

Key Points from the Editors

- Harassment in healthcare settings is often underrecognized and can cause significant physical and psychological harm. It negatively impacts both the well-being of healthcare workers and the quality of patient care.
- There has been an increase in violence directed at healthcare workers, particularly in emergency departments. The COVID-19 pandemic exposed vulnerabilities in workplace culture, exacerbating harassment and violence in healthcare settings, specially against healthcare professionals.
- Both pregnant and childless professionals are vulnerable to harassment, bullying, and discrimination in the workplace, which negatively impacts the healthcare system.

Main Objectives

After reading this chapter, you will be able to:

- Distinguish between harassment, bullying, and discrimination, and understand how they manifest in perioperative and critical care settings.
- Identify the risk factors that make perioperative and critical care environments particularly vulnerable to harassment and burnout.
- Evaluate strategies and proposed measures to improve working conditions and institutional support within these settings.

14.1 Introduction

For further reading in this chapter, it is essential to distinguish between the definitions of harassment, bullying, and discrimination. The differences in these definitions are linked to their legal consequences, as harassment is prohibited by various anti-discrimination laws [1].

1. Harassment:
   - The United Nations Entity for Gender Equality and the Empowerment of Women defines harassment as: "Any improper and unwelcome conduct that

might reasonably be expected or be perceived to cause offense or humiliation to another person." [2] Harassment can take many forms, and its classification is not always clear-cut. Within the workplace, the Advisory, Conciliation, and Arbitration Service categorizes harassment into three prongs [3]:
   (i) Harassment affiliated with "protected characteristics" (a person's socio-demographic information).
   (ii) Sexual harassment—unwelcomed or offensive sexual behavior that is recurrent or severe enough to cause harm or that involves implicit or explicit promises of favorable treatment or threats of adverse consequences.
   (iii) Harassment following a person's reaction to previous harassment.
2. Bullying:
   - The Advisory, Conciliation, and Arbitration Service defines it as: "Offensive, intimidating, malicious or insulting behavior, an abuse or misuse of power through means intended to undermine, humiliate, denigrate, or injure the recipient" [4].
3. Discrimination:
   - Unfair or prejudicial treatment of individuals based on attributes such as race, age, sexual orientation, disability, employment status, or political beliefs.

Perioperative and critical care medicine (CCM) often occurs in highly impersonal environments, with high levels of noise and light pollution, minimal privacy, and often lacking adequate staff relaxation areas. The perioperative and critical care setting is characterized by a high turnover of patients, with no pauses or interruptions in service delivery. Hospital administrations often perceive these specialties as indirectly productive and high cost, both in terms of personnel and medical supplies. Within CCM, staff (especially women and minorities) are constantly at an increased risk of burnout syndrome (BOS), harassment, and bullying due to various factors, which include compassion fatigue, interpersonal challenges with colleagues, management of life-threatening illnesses, and continual exposure to end-of-life issues [5, 6]. This chapter outlines the specific challenges faced by ICU staff, including ***gender-based harassment, bullying, and discrimination***. Improvements, preventive measures, and strategies will be addressed.

14.2 Prevalence of Harassment Against Healthcare Staff

The prevalence of workplace violence has been linked to increased rates of depression, burnout, moral distress, and suicidal ideation, all of which detrimentally affect workplace well-being and compromise clinical care and patient outcomes.

In a 2016 investigation conducted in the United Kingdom by the Royal College of Obstetricians and Gynaecologists, which involved 664 consultants, 44% of participants indicated they had been bullied by senior-level staff. Over 50% of respondents reported that such incidents occurred in more than half of their interactions with the aggressors. More than half of those surveyed also stated that the bullying

Harassment in healthcare settings is often vastly underestimated. It is crucial to recognize that workplace bullying and harassment can cause immediate, medium-term, or long-lasting physical and psychological harm. These behaviors pose serious risks to the health and safety of victims, manifesting as both direct and indirect threats.

hurt patient care. When inquired about whether the issue had been addressed, a striking 73% of respondents reported that it had not been adequately confronted [7].

While many countries have enacted laws to protect healthcare workers from discrimination and abuse, harassment against female providers persists. A survey conducted in 2021, which included approximately 629 intensive care nurses in Australia and New Zealand (67.7% female), revealed concerning statistics regarding workplace harassment [8] Within the past 12 months, 57.1% of participants reported having experienced bullying, with 59.6% of these incidents attributed to other nursing staff as the aggressors. Furthermore, 32.6% of respondents indicated they had faced discrimination, of which 51.7% was perpetrated by their nursing colleagues. Additionally, 1.9% of participants reported incidents of sexual harassment, with 34.6% of these occurrences involving male patients who inappropriately touched female staff during nursing interventions. Notably, 66% of participants chose not to report these incidents, reflecting a significant lack of confidence in existing mediation and reporting processes [8].

Reflection Point Do you know the incidence of harassment experienced by healthcare professionals in your country or at your hospital? How is this information currently tracked, and is it measured effectively?

Who should be responsible for addressing and measuring harassment in the healthcare environment? Should it be the responsibility of individual units, hospital leadership, government bodies, or other stakeholders?

Even though, since 2017, the number of women enrolling in medical school in the USA has surpassed that of men, incidents of sexual abuse against women—often perpetrated by male superiors—continue to persist. Notably, the fields of surgery and nursing have experienced the emergence of a significant #MeToo movement within medicine. Women have reported instances of male advances accompanied by threats of withholding employment, career advancement, or opportunities for personal growth, highlighting a pervasive culture of impunity among men in positions of power. As a result, many women often hesitate to report these incidents [9].

Reflection Point Why do women healthcare professionals often hesitate to report harassment in the workplace? Is it due to fear of retaliation, concerns about being labeled as troublemakers, or a lack of confidence in the reporting systems? What steps can be taken to overcome these barriers and ensure a safer, more equitable work environment for women?

14.3 Intersection of Harassment Against CCM Providers and Patient Care

There has been a concerning rise in violence against healthcare workers by patients and their families, particularly in emergency departments (EDs). A recent article in *The Journal of the American Medical Association (JAMA)* investigated the underlying causes of violent assaults against healthcare personnel. Prolonged waiting times, high service costs, and diminished availability of healthcare staff are factors that may contribute to this type of violence [10] This highlights how institutional hurdles that impact patients' healthcare experience may influence rates of harassment against staff.

In Italy, what was initially viewed as a phenomenon confined to areas of pronounced social distress has now begun to proliferate across a variety of settings [11] Numerous hospitals have initiated public awareness campaigns addressing this critical issue. However, no universally applicable models for fundamentally resolving the problem appear to be forthcoming. The repercussions of this situation include a diminished affinity for work environments in hospitals and a gradual alienation from such workplaces.

Close examination of these interactions reveals a toxic culture that undermines teamwork and erodes morale, ultimately jeopardizing patient care and the well-being of all staff involved. Each layer of aggression perpetuates a cycle of disrespect that not only impacts individual job satisfaction but also detracts from the collaborative spirit essential for effective healthcare delivery.

14.4 Difficulties During Pregnancy and Parenthood Related to Harassment

The structural shortage of healthcare professionals complicates the ability to secure temporary replacements during maternity leave. As a result, the increased workload typically falls on remaining staff, leading to extended overtime hours. A common sentiment expressed, especially toward female staff, is the expectation that others will "work in her place." This issue predominantly affects essential services, such as operating theatres and intensive care units (ICUs) [12], where operations cannot be reduced or paused. Consequently, despite legal entitlements in many countries, there is a notably low uptake of paternity leave.

A survey among European anesthesiologists and intensivists (including 3590 participants) indicated that only 41.4% of female respondents deemed their working conditions during pregnancy satisfactory; many expressed a desire to change roles due to concerns about workplace safety [13]. A qualitative study among American emergency medicine female physicians found that discrimination relating to "pregnancy/maternity leave" constituted 15.9% of harassment-related experiences, the second largest category following "patronizing behavior" [14].

The effects of harassment against physician mothers are critical to understand. A 2022 study surveyed a Physicians Moms online Facebook Group and found that two-thirds of participants had been victims of sexual harassment. Sexual harassment by patients in this group was associated with higher emotional exhaustion and patient depersonalization. WSH by colleagues was also associated with higher emotional exhaustion. Lastly, the study cited that social connectedness with other physician-mothers was associated with an increased sense of personal accomplishment, which highlights the potential of social support groups in mitigating the effects of harassment among female physicians [15]. This data highlights the need for equitable institutional policies that protect physician mothers, while also emphasizing the potential role of support groups in offering additional support and empowerment. The challenges faced by LGBT+ individuals are not discussed in detail, as they are rapidly evolving and vary significantly between countries, ranging from tolerance and support to a complete lack of opportunities.

> Pregnant women as well as childless women can be harassed in the workplace for different reasons, and both need protection and support. Education should address both conditions. Men deciding to accept less traditional role of parenthood might be discriminated and marginalized. Culture changes are needed for the benefit of all employers and ultimately for the benefit of patients.

It is critical to acknowledge how discrimination against physician mothers also negatively impacts the medical system at large. The USA is witnessing female physicians leaving medicine, with 40% of women physicians going part-time or leaving medicine altogether within 6 years of completing their residency [16]. A major reason for this is the lack of child support and childcare resources in the USA. As childbearing activities also fall on women, female physicians often do not get the support they need from institutions to continue working [16]. One in three physician moms in the USA has reported being discriminated against for their breastfeeding needs or due to pregnancy [16]. Losing female physicians is not only exacerbating physician shortages but also compromises the quality of care delivered to patients.

14.5 Childless Not by Choice and the Discriminatory Behavior Observed in the Workplace

Individuals who do not have children often face significant discriminatory behavior within the workplace, which can be attributed to societal norms and systemic biases that prioritize parenthood as a marker of commitment and stability. The demanding nature of medical training and job responsibilities often discourages individuals, especially women, from having children. Many women in the field may even choose to leave the profession altogether due to these pressures. Furthermore, it suggests that institutions may not fully recognize or address these challenges. In simpler terms, the high demands of healthcare jobs, particularly for women, make it harder to pursue both a career and parenthood, some of them may even postpone pregnancy or decide of not having children [17].

On the other hand, research suggests that employers may harbor implicit biases against childless employees, viewing them as less reliable or committed due to the absence of familial responsibilities. This bias can manifest in biased performance evaluations, limited career advancement, and a diminished sense of belonging in the workplace. These systemic challenges can negatively impact both the mental well-being and career progression of childless individuals. Therefore, it is essential to critically examine workplace policies and cultural attitudes toward non-parent employees to promote a more inclusive and equitable work environment [18].

Reflection Point How are childless doctors perceived in your environment? Are they expected to take on more workload compared to their colleagues with children?

Institutional expectations and cultural attitudes toward non-parent doctors might influence their professional responsibilities, job satisfaction, and overall well-being. Do these perceptions create an equitable or biased work environment?

14.6 Lessons Learned Regarding Harassment from the COVID-19 Pandemic

The COVID-19 pandemic has highlighted significant vulnerabilities in the workplace culture, notably concerning harassment [19]. During the initial wave, rapid team mobilization often resulted in a challenging environment where staff from diverse backgrounds faced heightened stress without adequate support [19]. The absence of clear guidelines and a lack of preparedness led to rising tensions [20], increased workloads, and ineffective communication. The near-total absence of internationally shared guidelines, varying competencies, a general lack of preparedness, inconsistent vocabulary, and sometimes dismissive attitudes from ICU staff toward less experienced colleagues—amid a climate of widespread fear—resulted in high turnover rates, burnout syndrome (BOS), and numerous career departures post-pandemic caused by bullying and harassment [19].

The pandemic has underscored the importance of preparedness: presence of clear protocols and guidelines, education and training in crisis management, support systems, networks and effective communication, leadership, institutional policies, and availability of adequate resources and equipment. A clear understanding of the needs and challenges involved helps reduce stress and minimizes the risk of conflicts, harassment, and violence in the workplace.

14.7 The Role Societal and Organizational Politics in Shaping Sustainable Healthcare Systems

Healthcare systems make up a large part of national budgets. While there are calls for greater collaboration between policymakers and the scientific community to support evidence-based medicine, healthcare systems often use evidence selectively, focusing on areas with stronger data and neglecting those with less. Politics plays an important role in healthcare but can sometimes become too dominant. Although laws vary by country, the influence of "stakeholders" is not always neutral and can affect the balance of the system [21]. Scandals involving public healthcare procurement, especially in areas with high costs, like operating rooms, which are vulnerable to manipulation may affect public opinion and create tensions within the healthcare system.

Political fluctuations can impact healthcare systems and the work environment. People in poor health or with disabilities are often less likely to vote or engage in democratic processes. Historically, progressive policies sought to attract voters by supporting disadvantaged and low-income groups. However, in recent years, many countries have seen a rise in conservative and populist parties, which capitalize on increasing public distrust in government institutions [22]. This distrust may extend to the healthcare system, affecting communication with the public and patients.

On the other hand, the traditional hierarchy in healthcare, from medical students to attending physicians, can create power dynamics that contribute to the marginalization and harassment of minority groups, including women. For example, mistreatment of medical students by supervising physicians has been a longstanding issue in medicine, highlighting how such interactions can foster a toxic workplace culture [23]. The AAMC recently found that one in three medical students and residents experienced mistreatment by faculty, and most chose not to report it [24]. Reports detailing the mistreatment of medical students are decade-spanning and range from verbal abuse to public humiliation, sexist comments, and more. Gender-based stereotypes and discrimination are also undoubtedly reflected in such mistreatment. A study that interviewed 10 medical students in Australia revealed that all 7 female respondents felt that gender overshadowed the quality of their clinical education [23]. This manifested in being offered fewer career-advancing opportunities and being ignored by male supervisors [23].

> When harassment and gender discrimination are seen as a normal part of medical training, something that students or new doctors are expected to endure, it fosters a workplace culture that tolerates ongoing harassment, particularly against female physicians.

Critical care environments, such as intensive care units (ICUs) and operating theatres, bring together healthcare professionals from all levels of competency to work closely together. These settings often foster "hierarchical violence," where accumulated frustrations at higher levels of the hierarchy lead to aggression toward lower-level staff [25]. Directors' frustrations may be directed at physicians, who, in turn, may display hostility toward nurses. Nurses, under their own pressures, may shift blame onto auxiliary staff, escalating frustrations further down the hierarchy, even reaching cleaning and maintenance workers. This creates a harmful cycle of blame and disrespect, devaluing the roles and expertise of individuals at all levels. These interactions contribute to a toxic work culture that undermines teamwork, erodes morale, and ultimately jeopardizes both patient care and staff well-being. The ongoing cycle of aggression and disrespect negatively affects job satisfaction and weakens the collaborative spirit necessary for effective healthcare delivery.

Reflection Point Have you personally witnessed or experienced "hierarchical violence" in healthcare settings? How did it impact your work and the overall team dynamics? Do you think that you have enough tools to recognize this form of harassment? What changes could help reduce these tensions and foster a more respectful and collaborative environment?

14.8 Potential Improvements

As discussed in this chapter, strategies fall under the purview of political decision-makers, whose perspectives can vary significantly depending on national contexts and educational systems.

1. **Combating Burnout:**
   (a) The European Society of Intensive Care Medicine (ESICM) has developed the "Hello Bundle" intervention aimed at reducing burnout among healthcare workers (HCWs) in intensive care units (ICUs) by promoting positive social interactions and fostering a supportive work atmosphere [26]. The forthcoming results of the "Hello" trial are anticipated to yield insights into effective strategies for mitigating burnout in ICU environments.
   (b) Raising awareness among emergency department staff about violence against healthcare workers is a crucial first step in addressing this issue. Providing tools for risk assessment can help prevent such incidents. For instance, utilizing resources like the Bröset Violence Checklist [27] enables early intervention in potential danger scenarios. Furthermore, investing in public awareness campaigns may prove more effective than merely allocating funds to address the problem reactively.
2. **Improving Clinical Environment:**
   (a) Increasing the flexibility of ICU bed usage allows for transitioning from intermediate care during non-critical periods to intensive care during critical phases. However, this shift still necessitates additional doctors and nurses to maintain appropriate patient-to-staff ratios (e.g., one nurse is needed for every two ICU beds, and one doctor for every eight beds) [28].

   (b) Doctors and nurses often feel observed and struggle to treat patients in the presence of their families. However, after an adjustment period, this environment typically becomes more comfortable and relaxed [29]. Nurses can foster stronger relationships with patients through their families, which may significantly reduce conflict levels and the likelihood of legal actions against healthcare professionals. Consequently, this organizational shift serves as an effective tool to mitigate both internal and external conflicts while promoting well-being in critical care settings [30]. Increasing literature suggests that extended access for family members to the ICU can benefit both them and the staff, without negatively impacting patient outcomes. A Brazilian randomized study found that the 12-month incidence of post-traumatic stress, anxiety, and depressive symptoms was lower among family members [31]. A systematic review published in Critical Care Medicine in 2018 confirmed that extended family visitation reduced patient anxiety and increased family satisfaction, with no correlation to ICU mortality, acquired infections, or prolonged stays [32].
   (c) CCM environments often feel impersonal, making it harder for patients to adapt. Healthcare staff in these settings need adequate rest and recovery to perform at their best. Workspace design plays a key role in staff well-being—environments with natural light, minimal noise, and relaxing views can reduce fatigue in ICUs. Designing human-centered spaces for both patients and staff can ease workloads and improve comfort [33]. Additionally, incorporating facilities like childcare and fitness areas into critical care areas is essential for staff well-being.
3. **Breaking the Medical Hierarchy:**
   (a) Health and politics should cooperate in a mutually reinforcing cycle. The expertise and insight of healthcare professionals provide a strong foundation for shaping health policies. Restoring public trust in democratic institutions starts with ensuring these institutions effectively address public needs, particularly in healthcare. Our aim is not to take a position, but to emphasize the significant impact that political elections can have on health policies, health disparities, and the importance of participating in the electoral process.
   (b) Institutional commitment to reducing harassment can include team-building initiatives that improve dynamics and enhance patient care. Examples are daily multidisciplinary meetings to clarify roles in critical care and perioperative settings, and debriefings after adverse events like cardiac arrests. These activities foster a supportive environment, promote teamwork, and help develop new skills [34, 35].
   (c) A reliable reporting system is essential in healthcare, especially in CCM, to protect staff and patients. Reporting adverse events, including near-misses, values everyone's input. However, doctors and nurses often hesitate to report due to fear of repercussions. Promoting transparency and collaboration, rather than blame, can foster a culture that accepts human error as part of daily practice [36, 37].

   (d) Low remuneration is a major challenge, especially in nursing. Adjusting salaries to reflect the cost of living and the increased workload and stress is a crucial political decision.
4. **Improving Psychosocial Well-Being.**
   (a) Despite widespread recommendations for psychological support services for CCM staff, these resources remain largely inaccessible. While clinical psychology services are sometimes offered to the families of critically ill patients, staff members often lack similar support. Although dedicated training in communication and conflict resolution is increasingly promoted by scientific societies, its uptake remains insufficient [38]. Team-building practices, such as meetings, social events (even outside of the hospital), and mindfulness activities, are now widely recognized—especially in high-pressure environments. When implemented, these practices can significantly improve teamwork and staff well-being.
   (b) Several observational studies have shown an association between compassionate, patient-centered care and improved clinical outcomes. Data suggests that healthcare professionals who consistently provide empathetic care experience less burnout, greater resilience, and better overall well-being. This challenges the conventional belief that emotionally investing in patients is burdensome and harmful. However, factors such as time constraints, lack of support, inadequate staffing, and limited resources often hinder clinicians' ability to deliver compassionate care [39–41].
   (c) A few patients leave the ICU completely recovered. The growing trend of post-ICU follow-up clinics offers a promising solution. Nurses and doctors reaching out to patients months after discharge—assessing their recovery, gathering feedback, and evaluating their critical care experience—can provide valuable "closure" for both patients and staff. This process helps reduce frustration and reinforces the effectiveness of specific treatments [42].
5. **Increasing Safety in Clinical Environments:**
   (a) The COVID-19 pandemic exposed significant disparities in ICU bed availability across countries and strained the relationship between healthcare workers and the public. In the USA, several states have introduced legislation to penalize those who aggress against healthcare professionals. For example, New Jersey passed the Health Care Heroes Violence Prevention Act in 2023, instituting stringent penalties for offenders. However, JAMA reports that enforcement of these laws remains limited, and the implementation of safety measures is often inadequate [43].

14.9 Conclusion

In conclusion, strategies for preventing harassment in healthcare settings focus on enhancing staff well-being, improving institutional recognition, and promoting professional development opportunities. Equally important is cultivating a culture of support and mutual respect within healthcare teams. The key to combating burnout lies not in escaping the pressures of critical care but in fostering connection—both at the bedside and within the team. Proactive measures, such as team-building activities, debriefing after adverse events, and ensuring adequate staffing levels, are crucial to reducing burnout and improving staff retention. Integrating family support into the ICU, implementing flexible visitation policies, and raising awareness of workplace violence are essential steps toward creating a more human-centered and supportive care environment. By prioritizing the well-being of healthcare workers, particularly in critical care settings, institutions can build a more resilient and effective workforce.

Proposed Actions

- Foster partnerships between policymakers and healthcare professionals to ensure health policies are informed by evidence and practical experience.
- Promote public engagement initiatives to rebuild trust in healthcare institutions and highlight the importance of participatory governance in health policy.
- Implement training programs aimed at breaking down traditional hierarchies in healthcare settings to mitigate harassment and encourage inclusivity among all staff levels.
- Establish mandatory reporting and support systems for staff to document and address mistreatment while promoting a non-punitive culture that values transparency.
- Adapt ICU designs to facilitate flexible patient care and enhance family visitation policies, leading to improved staff-patient relations and reduced conflict.
- Create more human-centered workspaces in clinical settings—promoting natural light, quiet areas, and spaces for relaxation—to support staff well-being.
- Enact and enforce legislation that addresses violence against healthcare workers while ensuring comprehensive safety measures are implemented in clinical settings.
- Evaluate and enhance risk assessment tools like the Bröset Violence Checklist to proactively identify and address potential threats to healthcare workers.

These action plans aim to shape a more supportive, effective, and equitable healthcare environment that considers the well-being of both staff and patients while addressing systemic issues in healthcare delivery.

References

1. GOV.UK. Discrimination: Your Rights. gov.uk. Published 2023. https://www.gov.uk/discrimination-your-rights
2. UN Women I UN System Coordination – Anti-harassment. www.un.org. https://www.un.org/womenwatch/uncoordination/antiharassment.html
3. ACAS. Harassment: Discrimination and the Equality Act 2010. Acas Published May 10, 2023. https://www.acas.org.uk/discrimination-and-the-law/harassment
4. ACAS. What bullying is: Bullying at work. ACAS. Published June 14, 2023. https://www.acas.org.uk/bullying-at-work
5. Cole SP, Siddiqui S. Well-being in the intensive care unit: looking beyond COVID-19. Anesthesiol Clin. 2022;40(2):373–82.
6. Boscolo A, Queirolo L, Navalesi P, the PADOVA Stress Group. The impact of psychophysiological wellbeing on executive functions among anaesthesia residents. Eur J Anaesthesiol. 2024; https://doi.org/10.1097/EJA.0000000000002106.
7. Shabazz T, Parry-Smith W, Oates S, Henderson S, Mountfield J. Consultants as victims of bullying and undermining: a survey of Royal College of Obstetricians and Gynaecologists consultant experiences. BMJ Open. 2016;6(6):e011462.
8. Parke R, Bates S, Carey M, Cavadino A, Ferguson A, Hammond N, Joyce F, Kirby S, Moeke-Maxwell T, Nona F, Mason K. Bullying, discrimination, and sexual harassment among intensive care unit nurses in Australia and New Zealand: an online survey. Aust Crit Care. 2023;36(1):10–8.
9. Chuck E. #MeToo in medicine: women, harassed in hospitals and operating rooms, await reckoning NBC News. (2018). https://www.nbcnews.com/storyline/sexual-misconduct/harassed-hospitals-operating-rooms-women-medicine-await-their-metoo-moment-n846031
10. Ninan RJ, Cohen IG, Adashi EY. State approaches to stopping violence against health care workers. JAMA. 2024;331(10):825–6.
11. Paterlini M. Italy toughens sanctions against perpetrators of violent attacks on hospital staff. BMJ. 2024;387:q2216. https://doi.org/10.1136/bmj.q2216.
12. Casilla-Lennon M, Hanchuk S, Zheng S, Kim DD, Press B, Nguyen JV, Grimshaw A, Leapman MS, Cavallo JA. Pregnancy in physicians: a scoping review. Am J Surg. 2022;223(1):36–46.
13. Zdravkovic M, Kabon B, Dow O, Klincová M, Bilotta F, Berger-Estilita J, Collaborators. Working conditions during pregnancy: a survey of 3590 European anaesthesiologists and intensivists. Br J Anaesth. 2024;133(5):1062–72. https://doi.org/10.1016/j.bja.2024.08.002.
14. Maso K, Theobald JL. Qualitative description of sexual harassment and discrimination of women in emergency medicine: giving the numbers a voice. AEM Educ Train. 2022;6(2) https://doi.org/10.1002/aet2.10727.
15. Linos E, Lasky-Fink J, Halley M, Sarkar U, Mangurian C, Sabry H, Linos E, Jagsi R. Impact of sexual harassment and social support on burnout in physician mothers. J Womens Health (Larchmt). 2022;31(7):932–40. https://doi.org/10.1089/jwh.2021.0487.
16. Paturel A. Why women leave medicine. AAMC; 2019. https://www.aamc.org/news/why-women-leave-medicine
17. Verniers C. Behind the maternal wall: the hidden backlash toward childfree working women. J Theor Soc Psychol. 2020;4(3):107–24. https://doi.org/10.1002/jts5.65.
18. https://www.personneltoday.com/hr/childless-employee-edi-unseen-minority/
19. Feeley T, Ffrench-O'Carroll R, Tan MH, Magner C, L'Estrange K, O'Rathallaigh E, Whelan S, Lyons B, O'Connor E. A model for occupational stress amongst paediatric and adult critical care staff during COVID-19 pandemic. Int Arch Occup Environ Health. 2021;94(7):1721–37.
20. Kira IA, Shuwiekh HAM, Ashby JS, Elwakeel SA, Alhuwailah A, Sous MSF, Baali SBA, Azdaou C, Oliemat EM, Jamil HJ. The impact of COVID-19 traumatic stressors on mental health: is COVID-19 a new trauma type. Int J Ment Health Addict. 2023;21(1):51–70.
21. World Health Organization. The impact of COVID-19 on health and care workers: a closer look at deaths. World Health Organization. (2021). https://iris.who.int/handle/10665/345300

22. Brubaker L, Curfman G, Ross JS, Bibbins-Domingo K. Health and the 2024 US election. *JAMA* Published online October 21, 2024. https://doi.org/10.1001/jama.2024.21511, 1791.
23. Colenbrander L, Causer L, Haire B. If you can't make it, you're not tough enough to do medicine': a qualitative study of Sydney-based medical students' experiences of bullying and harassment in clinical settings. BMC Med Educ. 2020;20(1):86. https://doi.org/10.1186/s12909-020-02001-y.
24. (2024) Medical schools work to end student mistreatment. In: AAMC.
25. Bass GA, Chang CWJ, Winkle JM, Cecconi M, Kudchadkar SR, Akuamoah-Boateng K, Einav S, Duffy CC, Hidalgo J, Rodriquez-Vega GM, Gandra-d'Almeida AJ, Barletta JF, Kaplan LJ. In-hospital violence and its impact on critical care practitioners. Crit Care Med. 2024;52(7):1113–26. https://doi.org/10.1097/CCM.0000000000006189.
26. Azoulay E, Barnes NK, Nainan-Myatra S, Delgado MM, Arabi Y, Boulanger C, Mistraletti G, Theodorakopoulou M, Van Heerden V, Paiva JA, Demirkýran O, La Calle GH, Al Fares A, Burghi G, Francois G, Barth A, De Waele J, Jaber S, Darmon M, Cecconi M. HELLO: a protocol for a cluster randomized controlled trial to enhance interpersonal relationships and team cohesion among ICU healthcare professionals. Intensive Care Med Exp. 2024;12(1):90. https://doi.org/10.1186/s40635-024-00677-w.
27. Woods P, Almvik R. The Brøset violence checklist (BVC). Acta Psychiatr Scand Suppl. 2002;412:103–5. https://doi.org/10.1034/j.1600-0447.106.s412.22.x.
28. Gjessing K, Steindal SA, Kvande ME. Collaboration between nurses and doctors in the decision-making process when considering ending the life-prolonging treatment of intensive care patients. Nurs Open. 2023;10(1):306–15. https://doi.org/10.1002/nop2.1305.
29. Schwartz AC, Dunn SE, Simon HFM, Velasquez A, Garner D, Tran DQ Jr, Kaslow NJ. Making family-centered care for adults in the ICU a reality. Front Psych. 2022;13:837708. https://doi.org/10.3389/fpsyt.2022.837708.
30. Scott P, Thomson P, Shepherd A. Families of patients in ICU: a scoping review of their needs and satisfaction with care. Nurs Open. 2019;6(3):698–712. https://doi.org/10.1002/nop2.287.
31. de Souza JMB, Miozzo AP, da Rosa M, Dos Santos R, Mocellin D, Rech GS, Trott G, GPM E, Sganzerla D, de Souza D, Rosa RG, Teixeira C. Long-term effects of flexible visitation in the intensive care unit on family members' mental health: 12-month results from a randomized clinical trial. Intensive Care Med. 2024;50(10):1614–21.
32. Nassar Junior AP, Besen BAMP, Robinson CC, Falavigna M, Teixeira C, Rosa RG. Flexible versus restrictive visiting policies in ICUs: a systematic review and meta-analysis. Crit Care Med. 2018;46(7):1175–80.
33. Rapport F, Francis-Auton E, Cartmill J, Ryder T, Braithwaite J, Clay-Williams R. A mobile methods pilot study of surgical spaces: 'fit for purpose? Organisational productivity and workforce wellbeing in workspaces in hospital' (FLOURISH). BMC Health Serv Res. 2020;20(1):78. https://doi.org/10.1186/s12913-020-4938-8.
34. Buljac-Samardzic M, Doekhie KD, van Wijngaarden JDH. Interventions to improve team effectiveness within health care: a systematic review of the past decade. Hum Resour Health. 2020;18(1):2. https://doi.org/10.1186/s12960-019-0411-3.
35. https://www.apsf.org/article/teamwork-in-the-operating-room-an-essential-for-patient-safety/
36. Staender S. Incident reporting in anaesthesiology. Best Pract Res Clin Anaesthesiol. 2011;25(2):207–14. https://doi.org/10.1016/j.bpa.2011.01.005.
37. Wehkamp K, Kuhn E, Petzina R, Buyx A, Rogge A. Enhancing patient safety by integrating ethical dimensions to critical incident reporting systems. BMC Med Ethics. 2021;22(1):26. https://doi.org/10.1186/s12910-021-00593-8.
38. Ricou B, Gigon F, Durand-Steiner E, Liesenberg M, Chemin-Renais C, Merlani P, Delaloye S. Initiative for burnout of ICU caregivers: feasibility and preliminary results of a psychological support. J Intensive Care Med. 2020;35(6):562–9. https://doi.org/10.1177/0885066618768223.
39. Siddiqui S, Mohamed E, Subramaniam B, Orui H, Nurok M, Cobas MA, Nunnally ME, Hartog C, Gillon R, Lown BA. Intensivists' perceptions of what is missing in their compassionate care during interactions in the intensive care unit. BMC Health Serv Res. 2022;22(1):1188. https://doi.org/10.1186/s12913-022-08584-0.

40. Siddiqui S, Hartog C. Drivers and drainers of compassion in intensive care medicine: an empirical study using video vignettes. PLoS One. 2023;18(3):e0283302. https://doi.org/10.1371/journal.pone.0283302.
41. Barber S, Moreno-Leguizamon CJ. Can narrative medicine education contribute to the delivery of compassionate care? A review of the literature. Med Humanit. 2017;43(3):199–203. https://doi.org/10.1136/medhum-2017-011242.
42. Zhang RX, Xu Y, Tian Y, He L, Chu Y. ICU follow-up services and their impact on post-intensive care syndrome: a scoping review protocol. BMJ Open. 2024;14(11):e089824. https://doi.org/10.1136/bmjopen-2024-089824.
43. Ninan RJ, Cohen IG, Adashi EY. State approaches to stopping violence against health care workers. JAMA. 2024;331(10):825–6. https://doi.org/10.1001/jama.2024.1140.

Cross-section of Today: Current Scenarios and Actions Taken to Promote Diversity, Equality and Inclusivity in the Workplace

15

Mia Gisselbaek and Sarah Saxena

Key Points from the Editors

- Gender equity in critical care and perioperative medicine is often hindered by subtle, unconscious barriers built into the system, such as implicit biases, societal expectations, and a lack of women's self-confidence.
- National and international organizations are taking steps to promote gender equity in these fields, focusing on policy changes, mentorship programs, increased research funding, and creating a supportive environment for women.
- More qualitative research is needed to explore the barriers women face in reaching leadership positions. While data on women's representation is available, there is a lack of insight into the reasons behind their underrepresentation, which is crucial for developing effective strategies to improve equity.

Supplementary Information The online version contains supplementary material available at https://doi.org/10.1007/978-3-031-86286-1_15.

M. Gisselbaek
Division of Anesthesiology, Department of Anesthesiology, Pharmacology, Intensive Care, and Emergency Medicine, Geneva University Hospitals and Faculty of Medicine, University of Geneva, Geneva, Switzerland

Unit of Development and Research in Medical Education (UDREM), Faculty of Medicine, University of Geneva, Geneva, Switzerland

S. Saxena (✉)
Department of Anesthesiology, Helora, Mons, Belgium

Department of Surgery, UMons, Research Institute for Health Sciences and Technology, University of Mons, Mons, Belgium

V. Neskovic, F. Rubulotta (eds.), *Diversity, Gender Equity and Inclusion in Critical Care and Perioperative Medicine*,
https://doi.org/10.1007/978-3-031-86286-1_15

Main Objectives

After reading this chapter, you will be able to:

- Explain key barriers to women's career progression in critical care and perioperative medicine, including implicit and explicit bias, the "leaky pipeline" phenomenon, the role of intersectionality, organizational weaknesses (such as rigid work structures and hours), and the lack of mentorship or family support.
- Categorize international initiatives aimed at advancing gender equity in healthcare, with a focus on critical care and perioperative medicine.
- Differentiate between institutional and individual efforts to raise awareness of gender equity challenges and explore potential solutions.

15.1 Introduction: Key Challenges to Gender Equity

The quest for gender equity in critical care and perioperative medicine is a multifaceted challenge that requires a comprehensive understanding of the barriers faced by women in these demanding fields. While there have been notable advancements in institutional policies and cultural shifts, many systemic challenges remain.

This chapter explores the various obstacles to achieving gender equity, including implicit and explicit biases, the "leaky pipeline" phenomenon, work-life balance issues, and the lack of family-friendly policies. Additionally, it highlights the international actions being taken to address these challenges and emphasizes the importance of collaborative efforts in promoting gender equity across the globe.

15.2 Barriers to Gender Equity (Fig. 15.1)

15.2.1 Implicit and Explicit Bias

Implicit biases are among the most pervasive barriers to gender equity in critical care and perioperative medicine. These biases are often unconscious and can significantly affect decision-making processes, leading to disparities in recruitment, promotion, and professional recognition. Women are frequently perceived as less competent or less capable of handling leadership roles in high-stress environments, resulting in fewer opportunities for advancement.

A 2018 study on gender inequity in medicine found that implicit biases contribute significantly to the underrepresentation of women in senior positions [1]. Decision-makers, both male and female, often unconsciously favour male candidates for leadership roles [2]. This bias not only affects hiring decisions but also impacts the evaluation of women's competencies, leading to a lack of confidence in their abilities and potential.

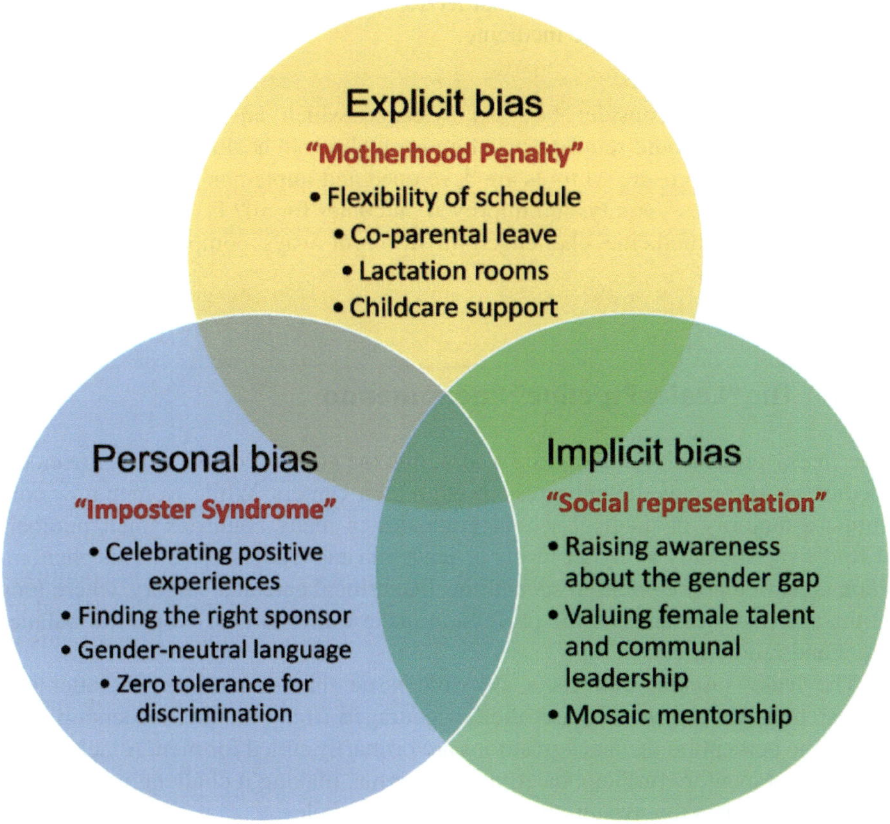

Fig. 15.1 Suggestions to overcome explicit, implicit, and personal bias. (Image reproduced with permission [2])

Moreover, explicit biases, which involve conscious attitudes and beliefs about gender roles, can further complicate the landscape for women in critical care and perioperative medicine. These biases manifest in various ways, from direct discrimination in hiring practices to the subtle undermining of women's authority in clinical settings. The combination of implicit and explicit biases creates a challenging environment for women, making it difficult for them to assert their leadership and expertise.

A new concern in this regard is the role artificial intelligence (AI) plays in perpetuating these biases. AI systems used in healthcare often reflect societal stereotypes, which can reinforce the misrepresentation of anaesthesiologists and intensivists as predominantly male [3]. Whether through biased training data or algorithms that overrepresent men in these roles, AI can inadvertently perpetuate the belief that leadership and expertise in these fields belong primarily to men. This technological bias, layered onto existing implicit and explicit prejudices, further marginalizes women and makes it harder for them to be recognized as leaders in critical care and perioperative medicine.

Reflection Point Consider how AI systems, which are often trained on historical data, could reinforce existing inequalities in healthcare. What steps can be taken to ensure AI tools are developed and implemented in a way that promotes fairness, equity, and improved outcomes for all? Is critical care and perioperative medicine challenged in different ways compering to other medical fields?

15.3 The "Leaky Pipeline" Phenomenon

The "leaky pipeline" is a term used to describe the gradual loss of women from the medical workforce as they progress through their careers. While women now constitute a majority of medical school graduates in many countries, their numbers dwindle significantly at higher levels of academia and leadership [2]. This phenomenon is particularly evident in specialities like critical care and surgery, where long hours and high demands of the profession make it difficult for women to balance work and family life.

The leaky pipeline reflects a systemic issue that requires urgent attention. Research shows that women are often discouraged from pursuing leadership roles due to the perception that such positions are primarily suited for men. A lack of role models and mentors further exacerbates this issue, making it challenging for aspiring female leaders to envision themselves in senior roles.

Compounding this is the impostor phenomenon, where women may doubt their abilities and fear being exposed as frauds, despite their qualifications [4]. This self-doubt, intensified by external biases, discourages many from pursuing leadership roles, further perpetuating gender disparities in critical care and perioperative medicine.

If you wish to learn more about **Impostor syndrome**, follow the link to a short video. The author of this chapter explains in single terms the meaning of the impostor syndrome and the importance of mentoring.

LEGEND OF THE VIDEO IS" IMPOSTOR SYNDROME AND THE ROLE OF MENTORSHIP".

As women advance in their careers, they face numerous challenges that contribute to their exit from high-demand specialities. The lack of flexible work options and support systems, such as childcare, exacerbates these challenges. Many women are forced to choose between their professional aspirations and familial responsibilities, leading to a significant drop in their representation in leadership roles [5, 6].

15.4 Work-Life Balance and Rigid Work Structures

The demanding nature of critical care and surgery presents additional challenges for women, particularly those with caregiving responsibilities. The lack of flexible working arrangements, long hours, and unpredictability of the work can make it challenging for women to balance their professional and personal lives [6]. This imbalance often leads to burnout or the decision to step away from high-demand specialities in favour of more flexible career paths.

In many cases, hospitals and medical institutions have not yet implemented sufficient family-friendly policies to accommodate the needs of female professionals. Onsite childcare, lactation rooms, parental leave, and flexible scheduling are essential components of a supportive work environment. Especially in anaesthesiology and critical care, the demanding nature of these roles makes it particularly challenging for female professionals to take time off for breastfeeding or lactation breaks, given the high level of responsibility and the unpredictable nature of the work. Without these resources, women may feel compelled to abandon their careers or pursue less demanding specialities.

Rigid work structures not only hinder women's career progression but also perpetuate the stereotype that caregiving responsibilities are primarily women's work. The expectation that women should fulfil these roles, combined with the demands of their professional duties, creates an untenable situation that can lead to feelings of guilt, inadequacy, and ultimately, attrition from the workforce.

> **Reflection Point** Rigid work structures and hours can hold back women's career growth. Is offering part-time work a solution? Does it end up reinforcing the idea that part-time jobs are for women, even when it's meant to make schedules more flexible? Are there other solutions?

15.5 Systemic Barriers to Leadership

Systemic barriers further contribute to the underrepresentation of women in leadership roles within critical care and perioperative medicine. Organizational cultures that prioritize traditional masculine traits, such as assertiveness and competitiveness, often marginalize women who may exhibit different leadership styles [7]. This cultural bias can create an environment where women feel undervalued and unsupported, discouraging them from seeking advancement.

Additionally, the lack of transparency in promotion processes can disadvantage women, as they may not be privy to the same networks and opportunities as their male counterparts. Women often find themselves excluded from informal discussions and networking opportunities, which can be crucial for career advancement. The absence of structured mentorship programs and leadership training further exacerbates these disparities, leaving women without the necessary tools to navigate the complexities of leadership in critical care and perioperative medicine [8].

15.6 The Role of Intersectionality

While gender is a significant factor in the quest for equity, it is essential to recognize the role of intersectionality in shaping women's experiences in critical care and perioperative medicine. Women of colour, those from lower socioeconomic backgrounds, and individuals from marginalized communities often face compounded challenges that exacerbate existing barriers to equity.

Research has shown that women from diverse backgrounds may experience higher levels of discrimination and bias, further hindering their professional growth. Addressing gender equity must therefore include a commitment to understanding and dismantling the intersecting systems of oppression that disproportionately affect women from diverse backgrounds [9].

Intersectionality in bullets: (Kimberlé Crenshaw—On Intersectionality—keynote—WOW 2016)

- **Intersectionality** is an analytical framework for understanding how a person's various social and political identities combine to create different modes of discrimination or privilege.
- In defining identities **gender, caste, sex, race, ethnicity, class, sexuality, religion, disability, weight, and physical appearance** may all combine, and it is usually not just the gender that enables bias, stereotypes and discrimination.
- Intersectionality may be **empowering and oppressing**, and both result in discrimination.

15.7 International Actions Towards Gender Equity

In response to these challenges, various national and international organizations have taken steps to promote gender equity in critical care and perioperative medicine. These actions focus on policy reform, mentorship programs, research funding, and creating a supportive environment for women in these fields.

15.8 Policy and Organizational Reforms

Several critical care organizations have implemented policies aimed at promoting diversity and inclusion. For instance, the World Federation of Intensive and Critical Care (WFICC) and the European Society of Intensive Care Medicine (ESICM) have both adopted diversity and inclusion policies that call for equal representation of women in leadership and decision-making roles [10, 11]. These policies serve as a framework for fostering a more inclusive environment and addressing the systemic barriers that have historically hindered women's advancement.

In North America, the Society of Critical Care Medicine (SCCM) has introduced various initiatives aimed at addressing gender disparities [12]. The SCCM's Diversity, Equity, and Inclusion (DEI) Task Force has been actively working to implement gender-sensitive policies and ensure that women are represented in all levels of decision-making, from task forces to executive committees. By prioritizing diversity in leadership, these organizations aim to create a more equitable and inclusive landscape for all healthcare professionals.

15.9 Mentorship and Sponsorship Programs

Mentorship and sponsorship are critical tools for promoting gender equity in medicine. Recognizing this, several organizations have launched mentorship programs specifically designed to support women in critical care and perioperative medicine. These programs connect female professionals with senior mentors who provide guidance, support, and career development opportunities.

For example, in the United States, programs like Women in Critical Care (WIN ANZICS) provide networking and mentorship opportunities for female intensivists [13]. These programs also work to raise awareness about the importance of diversity in critical care teams and the role of women in advancing the field. By fostering connections between experienced leaders and emerging professionals, mentorship programs play a crucial role in empowering women to take on leadership positions.

In Europe, organizations like the ESICM have also developed successful mentorship programs that provide female healthcare professionals with access to senior leaders who can advocate for their advancement [14]. These programs emphasize the importance of sponsorship, where senior mentors not only guide but actively promote women's careers by nominating them for leadership positions, awards, and speaking engagements. Research has shown that mentorship can significantly impact women's career trajectories, helping them overcome barriers and build the confidence needed to pursue leadership roles.

15.9.1 Mentorship for Women by Women

Mentorship for women by women is a powerful strategy for promoting gender equity in critical care and perioperative medicine [8]. Female mentors provide invaluable guidance and support, helping emerging female professionals navigate the unique challenges they face in male-dominated environments. These mentorship relationships foster a sense of community and empowerment, enabling women to share experiences, gain confidence, and develop essential leadership skills. By connecting with seasoned professionals who understand the intricacies of gender bias and work-life balance, mentees can access tailored advice and encouragement that is often more relatable than traditional mentorship models. Furthermore, these relationships create networks that amplify women's voices and advocate for their advancement, ultimately leading to increased representation of women in leadership positions within healthcare. The reciprocal nature of mentorship also enriches mentors' careers, as they gain fresh perspectives and insights from the next generation of female leaders, fostering a culture of collaboration and support that can transform the workplace for women in medicine.

Reflection Point The idea that mentoring can enhance leadership skills is powerful. The more mentors actively engage in supporting others, the more they not only help their mentees but also grow their own confidence and leadership capabilities. Can mentoring relationships, particularly cross-gender ones (women mentoring men) play a role in reducing workplace inequality and promoting leadership development?

15.10 Research and Academic Initiatives

Addressing the gender gap in academic publishing and research is another critical focus of international efforts to promote gender equity. Studies have shown that women are significantly underrepresented as lead authors in critical care and perioperative medicine research, and they are less likely to receive research funding or awards compared to their male counterparts.

To address this, organizations like the SCCM and the Canadian Institutes of Health Research (CIHR) have implemented gender-sensitive research policies that ensure equitable access to research funding and opportunities [15]. Additionally, many international conferences on critical care now include sessions on gender diversity, where participants discuss best practices for promoting gender equity in research. By fostering an environment where women are encouraged to contribute to research, these organizations aim to close the gender gap and ensure that diverse perspectives are represented in medical literature.

The role of editorial boards in shaping the landscape of research publishing cannot be overlooked. Many journals have recognized the need for greater diversity among their editorial boards and have made concerted efforts to include more women in leadership positions. By ensuring that women have a voice in the editorial process, these journals can contribute to a more equitable publishing environment.

15.11 The Role of Global Conferences and Collaborations

Global conferences play a crucial role in advancing gender equity by providing platforms for discussion, collaboration, and knowledge sharing. Many critical care and perioperative medicine conferences now include dedicated sessions on gender diversity, equity, and inclusion. These sessions focus on sharing best practices, discussing challenges, and highlighting successful strategies for promoting gender equity. The number of women speakers at international conferences has steadily increased over the years, reflecting the success of efforts to promote gender equity and inclusion in the field [16].

By fostering international collaboration, these conferences help create a global movement towards gender equity in healthcare. Attendees can share their experiences, learn from one another, and develop actionable strategies for promoting gender equity within their own institutions and countries.

15.11.1 Day-Care Facilities at Medical Conferences

The presence of day-care facilities at medical conferences is a crucial step towards fostering an inclusive environment that supports the participation of healthcare professionals, particularly women, who often bear the brunt of caregiving responsibilities. By providing accessible childcare services, conferences enable parents to engage fully in educational sessions, networking opportunities, and discussions without the added stress of arranging alternative care for their children. Moreover, integrating children into the professional realm, even at a conference setting, serves as an invaluable opportunity to teach them about their parents' vital work as intensivists. This exposure not only cultivates respect and understanding for the healthcare profession but also instils a sense of pride in children as they witness firsthand the dedication and passion that their parents bring to their roles. Encouraging children to appreciate the complexities and significance of critical care can inspire future generations to consider careers in medicine, ultimately contributing to a more diverse and empathetic healthcare workforce.

15.12 Advocacy and Awareness Campaigns

Advocacy and awareness campaigns play a vital role in promoting gender equity by raising awareness about the challenges faced by women in critical care and perioperative medicine. Organizations such as the WFICC and the SCCM have launched campaigns aimed at highlighting the importance of gender equity in healthcare [11, 12].

These campaigns often feature personal stories from female healthcare professionals who have navigated the complexities of gender bias and discrimination. By sharing their experiences, these women inspire others to act and advocate for change. Furthermore, these campaigns aim to educate the broader medical community about the systemic barriers that hinder women's progress and promote a culture of inclusivity and support.

15.13 The Future of Gender Equity in Critical Care and Perioperative Medicine

Achieving gender equity in critical care and perioperative medicine requires a concerted effort from all stakeholders, including medical institutions, professional organizations, and individual practitioners. The progress made thus far should be acknowledged, but there is still much work to be done to dismantle the systemic barriers that perpetuate gender disparities.

15.14 The Importance of Leadership Commitment

Leadership commitment is essential for fostering a culture of gender equity within medical institutions. Senior leaders must actively advocate for gender equity, promote diversity in hiring and promotion practices, and implement family-friendly policies that support women's career advancement. By prioritizing gender equity at the organizational level, institutions can create an environment where women feel valued, supported, and empowered to pursue leadership roles.

15.15 The Role of Education and Training

Education and training programs play a crucial role in addressing gender bias and promoting awareness of the challenges faced by women in critical care and perioperative medicine. Incorporating training on implicit bias, diversity, and inclusion into medical education can help future healthcare professionals recognize and challenge their biases, leading to a more equitable environment.

Continuing medical education (CME) programs should also include modules focused on gender equity and leadership development for female professionals. By equipping women with the knowledge and skills needed to navigate the complexities of leadership, these programs can help bridge the gender gap in critical care and perioperative medicine.

15.16 Collaborative Efforts for Lasting Change

Collaboration among organizations, institutions, and individuals is vital for creating lasting change. By working together, stakeholders can share resources, knowledge, and best practices to promote gender equity. Collaborative initiatives can also amplify the voices of women in critical care and perioperative medicine, creating a collective movement for change.

International partnerships and alliances can enhance the visibility of gender equity initiatives and promote a global agenda for change. Organizations like the WFICC and ESICM should continue to collaborate with other global health organizations to share successful strategies and advocate for policies that promote gender equity.

15.17 Conclusion

The journey towards gender equity in critical care and perioperative medicine is complex and multifaceted, shaped by a myriad of cultural, institutional, and systemic factors. While significant challenges remain—ranging from implicit and explicit biases to a lack of support systems for work-life balance—concerted efforts at the international, national, and institutional levels can foster a more inclusive and equitable environment for women in these fields. By actively addressing the root causes of gender disparities, such as dismantling systemic barriers that hinder women's professional advancement and promoting mentorship programs that empower female professionals, we can create pathways for their success.

In addition, there is a critical need for qualitative research to better understand the underlying barriers women face in reaching leadership roles [17]. By gaining deeper insights into the specific experiences and challenges encountered by female professionals, researchers can inform more effective strategies for promoting gender equity and inclusivity. Continued research on gender-sensitive practices is essential, along with advocacy for policy reforms that address these structural issues.

As we move forward, it is crucial to recognize the importance of intersectionality, acknowledging that the experiences of women in medicine are not monolithic. Women of different backgrounds, ethnicities, and socioeconomic statuses face unique challenges that must be addressed to achieve true equity. By amplifying the voices of women from all walks of life and fostering a culture of inclusivity within the healthcare system, we can ensure that diverse perspectives are valued and that solutions are tailored to meet the varied needs of all practitioners.

Furthermore, educational institutions and professional organizations must commit to ongoing training and awareness programs that address gender bias and cultivate an environment of respect and equality. As we advocate for policies that support family-friendly work environments, we also pave the way for future generations of healthcare professionals who can thrive without compromising their personal lives.

The time for action is now; the momentum for change is building, and together, we can ensure that gender equity becomes a reality in critical care and perioperative medicine. By fostering collaborative efforts, engaging in open dialogue, and prioritizing gender equity in all levels of decision-making, we can build a more equitable healthcare system that not only benefits women but enhances the quality of care for patients. The commitment to this cause will ultimately pave the way for a future where women can flourish in their careers, become leaders in their fields, and inspire the next generation of healthcare professionals to continue the pursuit of equality in medicine.

Proposed Actions

- Foster collaboration across organizations, institutions, and individuals to create sustainable change. Share resources, knowledge, and best practices to advance gender equity in critical care and perioperative medicine. Amplify the voices of women in these fields to build a sustainable change.
- Develop and support mentorship and sponsorship programs to encourage gender equity in critical care and perioperative medicine. Connect female professionals with experienced mentors who can offer guidance, support, and career development opportunities.
- Make day-care facilities mandatory at medical conferences and scientific events to support healthcare professionals—especially women—who often bear the burden of caregiving responsibilities. Encourage the participation of women by ensuring childcare options are available and accessible.

References

1. Abdellatif W, Ding J, Jalal S, et al. Leadership gender disparity within research-intensive medical schools: a transcontinental thematic analysis. J Contin Educ Health Prof. 2019;39(4):243–50. https://doi.org/10.1097/CEH.0000000000000270.
2. Gisselbaek M, Barreto Chang O, Saxena S. Gender equity in anesthesia: is it time to rock the boat? BMC Anesthesiol. 2023;23(1):67. https://doi.org/10.1186/s12871-023-01987-4.
3. Gisselbaek M, Köselerli E, Suppan M, et al. Gender bias in images of anaesthesiologists generated by artificial intelligence. Br J Anaesth. 2024;133(3):692–5. https://doi.org/10.1016/j.bja.2024.05.027.
4. Gisselbaek M, Hontoir S, Pesonen AE, et al. Impostor syndrome in anaesthesiology primarily affects female and junior physicians. Br J Anaesth. 2024;132(2):407–9. https://doi.org/10.1016/j.bja.2023.09.025.
5. Carter JC, Purcell N, Stewart CH, Pearce GC, Balkin M, Allen KJ. Still a "boys" club': a qualitative analysis of how gender affects a career in anaesthesia in Australia and Aotearoa New Zealand. Anaesthesia. 2024;79(7):694–705. https://doi.org/10.1111/anae.16281.
6. Allen KJ, Chiavaroli N, Reid KJ. Successful return to work in anaesthesia after maternity leave: a qualitative study. Anaesthesia. 2024;79(7):706–14. https://doi.org/10.1111/anae.16231.
7. Winkel AF, Telzak B, Shaw J, et al. The role of gender in careers in medicine: a systematic review and thematic synthesis of qualitative literature. J Gen Intern Med. 2021;36(8):2392–9. https://doi.org/10.1007/s11606-021-06836-z.
8. Gisselbaek M, Marsh B, Soriano L, et al. Gender and race/ethnicity dynamics in anesthesiology mentorship: results of a European survey. BMC Anesthesiol. 2024;24(1):311. https://doi.org/10.1186/s12871-024-02692-6.
9. Garrick A, Johnson WD, Arendt SW. Breaking barriers: strategies for fostering inclusivity in the workplace. Int J Acad Res Bus Soc Sci. 2024;14(2):128–52.
10. Diversity. ESICM. Accessed 9 Oct 2024. https://www.esicm.org/the-esicm/diversity/
11. Our Policies. World Federations of Intensive and Critical Care. August 3, 2018. Accessed October 9, 2024. https://www.wficc.com/about-us/our-policies
12. SCCM | Diversity, Equity, and Inclusion. Society of Critical Care Medicine (SCCM) Accessed 9 Oct 2024. https://sccm.org/About-SCCM/Diversity-Equity-and-Inclusion
13. Women in Intensive Care (WIN ANZICS). ANZICS. Accessed October 9, 2024. https://www.anzics.org/women-in-intensive-care-win-anzics/

14. NEXT-Mentoring. ESICM. Accessed 9 Oct 2024. https://www.esicm.org/education/career-development/ice-mentoring/
15. Government of Canada CI of HR. Equity, Diversity and Inclusion in the Research System - CIHR. June 24, 2021. Accessed October 9, 2024. https://cihr-irsc.gc.ca/e/52543.html
16. Dymore-Brown LA, Ahluwalia A, Dangoisse C, et al. An update on gender disparity in critical care conferences. Crit Care Explor. 2024;6(4):e1075. https://doi.org/10.1097/CCE.0000000000001075.
17. Gisselbaek M, Hudelson P, Savoldelli GL. A systematic scoping review of published qualitative research pertaining to the field of perioperative anesthesiology. Can J Anesth/J Can Anesth. 2021;68(12):1811–21. https://doi.org/10.1007/s12630-021-02106-y.

Index

V. Neskovic, F. Rubulotta (eds.), *Diversity, Gender Equity and Inclusion in Critical Care and Perioperative Medicine*,
https://doi.org/10.1007/978-3-031-86286-1

GPSR Compliance

The European Union's (EU) General Product Safety Regulation (GPSR) is a set of rules that requires consumer products to be safe and our obligations to ensure this.

If you have any concerns about our products, you can contact us on ProductSafety@springernature.com

In case Publisher is established outside the EU, the EU authorized representative is:

Springer Nature Customer Service Center GmbH
Europaplatz 3
69115 Heidelberg, Germany

Batch number: 10726060

Printed by Printforce, the Netherlands